Achieving and Maintaining Accreditation for Nursing School Programs

A Comprehensive Guide

Keith A. Beaulieu

**Achieving and Maintaining Accreditation for Nursing School Programs:
A Comprehensive Guide**

Cover Photo courtesy of iStock (Stock photo ID:599696102)

Published by Keith A. Beaulieu

Cape51@yahoo.com

Printed in the United States of America

First Printing: December 2024

ISBN 978-1-7360792-2-5 (Paperback)

ISBN 978-1-7360792-3-2 (Hardback)

First edition, 2024

10 9 8 7 6 5 4 3 2 1

Acknowledgments

I want to thank the **Sue & Bill Gross School of Nursing** at the University of California Irvine, who, through my work, tested and refined some of the practices listed in this publication.

I would also like to thank all those I work with in the **Society for Simulation in Healthcare Accreditation Council** and the many reviewers with whom I collaborate; they are true professionals and champions for both accreditation and healthcare simulation.

Dedication

For my wife, who pushes me every day to be a better version of
myself than I was the day before.

Contents

Introduction

Accreditation is a cornerstone of nursing education, ensuring that nursing programs meet established standards of quality and rigor. For nursing schools, obtaining and maintaining accreditation is not just a regulatory requirement but a commitment to delivering the best possible education and preparing the next generation of healthcare professionals. Accreditation provides external validation of a program's curriculum, faculty, resources, and overall effectiveness, directly impacting students, faculty, and the communities they serve.

The importance of accreditation cannot be overstated. According to the *National League for Nursing* (NLN), accreditation ensures that nursing programs are aligned with industry standards and are prepared to deliver high-quality, competent nurses to meet the evolving demands of the healthcare sector. Attending an accredited nursing program is crucial for prospective students - accreditation directly impacts eligibility for licensure exams and access to federal financial aid. Additionally, employers across the healthcare industry often prefer and sometimes require graduates from accredited programs. In a recent *American Association of Colleges of Nursing (AACN)* survey, 85% of healthcare employers prioritized hiring nurses from accredited programs, highlighting the critical role accreditation plays in shaping the workforce.

Accreditation also assures the public that nursing programs uphold standards that ensure patient safety and care quality. As the healthcare landscape continues to evolve, the stakes of nursing education rise. According to the *U.S. Bureau of Labor Statistics*, registered nurse employment is projected to grow 6% from 2021 to 2031, faster than the average for all occupations. As the demand for skilled nurses grows, the pressure for nursing programs to provide exceptional education and produce highly trained professionals has never been greater. Accreditation ensures that nursing schools are equipped to meet these needs by establishing clear benchmarks for academic excellence and clinical competency.

However, achieving and maintaining accreditation is a complex, ongoing process that requires significant effort, planning, and collaboration. It involves meeting strict regulatory standards and engaging in continuous self-assessment and improvement. Nursing programs must demonstrate their ability to provide evidence-based, high-quality instruction, maintain a robust curriculum, and offer adequate resources to support faculty and students. A 2022 report from the *National Council of State Boards of Nursing* (NCSBN) revealed that 96% of nursing schools with accreditation reported higher graduation rates than non-accredited programs, showcasing the link between accreditation and student success.

The accreditation journey begins with a comprehensive self-study and a site visit from accrediting bodies. It culminates in submitting evidence and documentation to demonstrate compliance with standards. For example, the *Accreditation Commission for Education in Nursing* (ACEN) and the *Commission on Collegiate Nursing Education* (CCNE) set rigorous program benchmarks to evaluate curriculum content, faculty qualifications, student outcomes, and institutional support. The process can take several months to complete, depending on the size and complexity of the program. Still, it is an investment in the long-term success and credibility of the nursing school.

Even once accreditation is granted, nursing programs must remain committed to maintaining these standards through periodic reports, reaccreditation cycles, and ongoing quality improvement efforts. According to a 2021 *AACN* study, 72% of nursing programs reported facing challenges in maintaining accreditation due to limited resources or shifts in regulatory requirements, indicating the ongoing effort required to stay accredited. For example, the 10-year reaccreditation cycle typically involves an in-depth review of program outcomes, curriculum updates, and institutional changes. These ongoing evaluations help ensure nursing schools align

This book is designed to guide nursing school administrators, faculty, and accreditation specialists through achieving and sustaining accreditation for their programs. Whether preparing for your first accreditation review or looking for strategies to strengthen your program's compliance and quality, this guide will provide valuable insights into every step of the process. You will learn about the key standards and expectations set by accrediting bodies, best practices for preparing for accreditation, and effective strategies for ensuring long-term success.

Achieving and maintaining accreditation is no small feat, but it is a vital investment in the future of nursing education. By adhering to established standards and embracing continuous improvement, nursing programs can improve and enhance their accreditation status. As evidenced by the statistics and findings from accrediting organizations and industry surveys, accredited programs are better equipped to meet the needs of their students and the healthcare system at large. This book will serve as your roadmap to that success, providing you with the tools, knowledge, and practical advice needed to navigate the complexities of accreditation in nursing education.

Chapter 1
Understanding Accreditation in Nursing Education

Accreditation is the cornerstone of quality assurance in higher education, particularly in nursing. It is an objective measure of a program's commitment to providing quality education that meets the standards set by recognized accrediting bodies. Accreditation in nursing education is a rigorous and systematic process that involves evaluating multiple aspects of a program, from the curriculum and faculty qualifications to student outcomes and institutional support. This chapter will explore the essential role of accreditation, its benefits, the key accrediting bodies, and the process of achieving and maintaining accreditation in nursing schools.

1.1 The Importance of Accreditation in Nursing Education

Accreditation in nursing is essential for maintaining high standards of education that ultimately impact patient care and safety. The role of accreditation is not just regulatory but foundational to ensuring that nursing programs produce competent, skilled professionals capable of meeting the healthcare system's demands. Without accreditation, nursing programs risk operating outside established quality standards, affecting the program's credibility and graduates' employability.

In a study by the *National League for Nursing (NLN)*, 92% of healthcare employers stated that they preferred to hire nurses from accredited programs, recognizing that these programs are more likely to produce highly skilled professionals equipped to handle complex patient care scenarios (National League for Nursing, 2021). Accreditation ensures that nursing programs follow evidence-based teaching practices, promote critical thinking, and foster professional development. For students, attending an accredited nursing program is crucial for eligibility to sit for licensure exams, such as the NCLEX-RN (National Council Licensure Examination for Registered Nurses), and access to federal financial aid.

Moreover, accreditation has far-reaching implications for healthcare outcomes. A 2018 study published in the *Journal of Nursing Education and Practice* found that hospitals and healthcare institutions that employed graduates from accredited nursing programs reported lower rates of patient readmission, fewer medication errors, and improved overall patient satisfaction. These findings underscore the critical role that accredited nursing education plays in shaping the future of healthcare.

1.2 The Key Accrediting Bodies for Nursing Programs

There are two primary accrediting bodies for nursing education programs in the United States: The *Accreditation Commission for Education in Nursing* (ACEN) and the *Commission on Collegiate Nursing Education* (CCNE). Each organization has a distinct focus, though both aim to ensure quality education for nursing students.

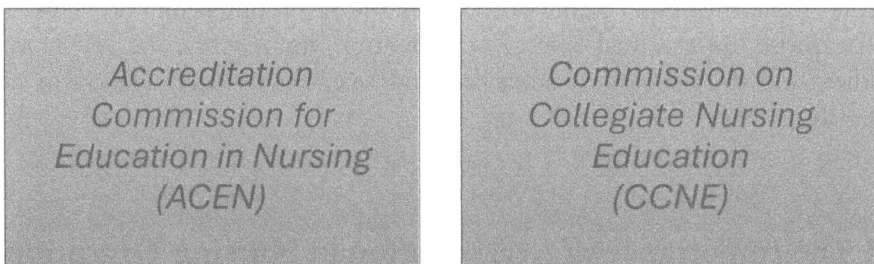

| Accreditation Commission for Education in Nursing (ACEN) | Commission on Collegiate Nursing Education (CCNE) |

Figure 1 Key Accrediting Bodies

The Accreditation Commission for Education in Nursing (ACEN)

ACEN is a nationally recognized accrediting body that accredits nursing programs at the associate, baccalaureate, master's, and doctoral levels. ACEN is one of the oldest accrediting bodies in nursing, with its roots going back to 1952. It provides accreditation for programs that aim to provide a sound education grounded in developing clinical skills, theoretical knowledge, and research-based practices.

The ACEN accreditation process evaluates the program's mission, resources, student learning outcomes, faculty qualifications, and effectiveness. Programs must demonstrate that they meet the organization's rigorous standards for curriculum content, student outcomes, and institutional support. ACEN accreditation ensures that nursing programs meet current standards of practice and the evolving healthcare delivery needs.

The Commission on Collegiate Nursing Education (CCNE)

The CCNE, a subsidiary of the *American Association of Colleges of Nursing* (AACN), accredits baccalaureate and graduate-level nursing programs. Established in 1996, CCNE has become one of the leading accrediting bodies in nursing education. It focuses on the quality of nursing education, including nursing schools' missions, objectives, and resources.

CCNE's standards strongly emphasize program outcomes, including graduation rates, licensure pass rates, and employment outcomes for graduates. This organization also evaluates the program's commitment to preparing students for professional roles in nursing and its ability to provide resources for both students and faculty. CCNE accreditation is widely recognized within the healthcare industry and a hallmark of excellence in nursing education.

1.3 Differences Between ACEN and CCNE

While ACEN and CCNE both serve the purpose of accrediting nursing programs, the primary difference lies in the types of programs they accredit and their focus. ACEN accredits nursing programs at all levels—associate, baccalaureate, and graduate—while CCNE primarily accredits baccalaureate and graduate-level programs. Additionally, CCNE emphasizes ensuring the program prepares students for leadership roles and advanced practice nursing. In contrast, ACEN focuses on the broader scope of nursing education at all levels.

The U.S. Department of Education recognizes accrediting bodies and ensures that nursing programs meet national standards. Many programs seek accreditation from both bodies to enhance their reputation and provide students with more significant opportunities.

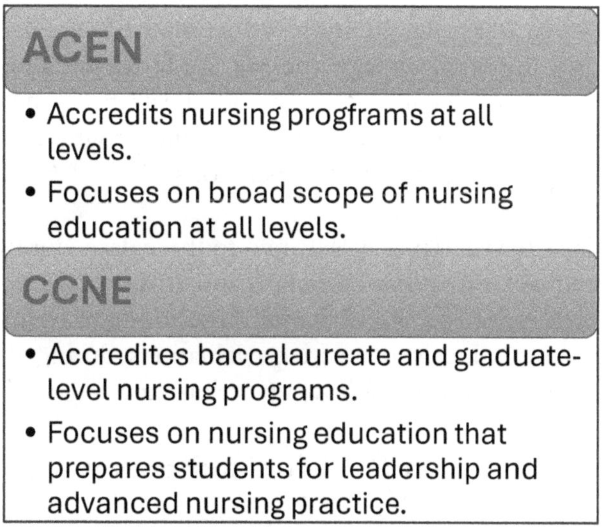

ACEN

- Accredits nursing progframs at all levels.
- Focuses on broad scope of nursing education at all levels.

CCNE

- Accredites baccalaureate and graduate-level nursing programs.
- Focuses on nursing education that prepares students for leadership and advanced nursing practice.

Figure 2 Accrediting Agency Differences

1.4 The Accreditation Process

Accreditation is a comprehensive and multi-step procedure. This section will outline the key steps in obtaining and maintaining accreditation for nursing programs.

Self-Study

The first step in the accreditation process is self-study. In this thorough internal evaluation, the nursing program assesses its strengths, weaknesses, and compliance with accrediting standards. During the self-study phase, programs review all aspects of their operation, including faculty qualifications, curriculum, student support services, and clinical placements. This process is essential for identifying areas for improvement and ensuring that the program is aligned with the standards set by accrediting bodies.

Comprehensive self-study is typically required several months before the accreditation visit. According to ACEN, 70% of nursing programs reported that conducting self-study was one of the most valuable components of the accreditation process, as it provided a roadmap for continuous improvement (ACEN, 2020).

Site Visit

After self-study, an evaluation team from the accrediting body conducts a site visit to assess the program's adherence to accreditation standards. During the site visit, the team reviews the self-study report, examines program materials, and meets with faculty, students, administrators, and clinical partners. This visit is crucial for gathering evidence of the program's effectiveness and ensuring its stated goals align with its operations.

The site visit typically lasts two to three days, during which the evaluators provide feedback on areas of strength and areas requiring improvement. For example, a 2021 report by the *American Association of Colleges of Nursing* found that 83% of programs received positive evaluations during the site visit, with most issues addressed through follow-up actions and ongoing support (AACN, 2021).

Accreditation Decision and Follow-Up

Following the site visit, the accrediting body will issue an accreditation decision, ranging from full accreditation to probationary status or denial. If a program is granted full accreditation, it typically remains accredited for 5 to 10 years, depending on the accrediting body's policies. However, suppose the program is granted probationary status. In that case, it must submit a follow-up report outlining how to address the identified deficiencies.

In some cases, programs denied accreditation can appeal the decision, providing additional evidence or making necessary adjustments to their operations. If the appeal is successful, the program may be granted provisional or full accreditation.

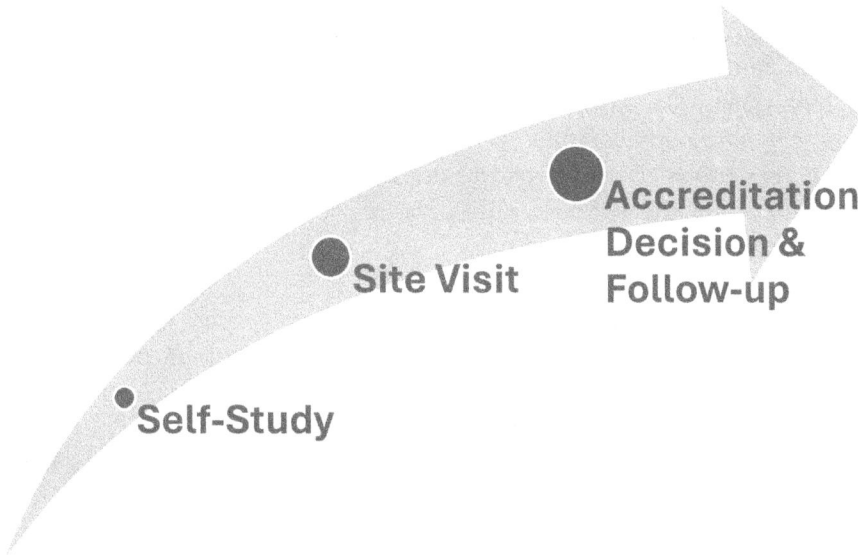

Accreditation
Decision &
Follow-up

Site Visit

Self-Study

Figure 3 The Accreditation Process

1.5 Maintaining Accreditation

Once a program has achieved accreditation, the work does not end. Maintaining accreditation requires continuous effort, including periodic self-assessment, documentation of program outcomes, and ongoing alignment with accrediting standards. Accreditation is typically granted for a specific period (usually 5–10 years), after which programs must undergo a reaccreditation process.

The reaccreditation process involves submitting updated documentation and undergoing another site visit, during which the program's performance is reassessed. Regular reporting is also required to demonstrate that the program continues to meet accreditation standards and address any areas of concern. Programs that fail to maintain accreditation risk losing eligibility for federal funding, impacting student enrollment and institutional reputation.

Additionally, many accrediting bodies require nursing programs to submit annual reports to track student outcomes, faculty qualifications, and other metrics. These reports allow the accrediting bodies to monitor ongoing compliance with standards and provide guidance for future improvements. For example, ACEN requires annual reports to demonstrate ongoing compliance with accreditation standards and provide updates on changes in the program's mission, faculty, and resources.

1.6 Benefits of Accreditation

Accreditation benefits nursing programs, students, and the broader healthcare system. For nursing schools, accreditation enhances institutional credibility, attracts high-quality faculty, and ensures that the program meets national standards. Attending an accredited program opens doors to licensure, financial aid, and career advancement opportunities for students. Most importantly, accreditation ensures that graduates are prepared to meet the complex demands of the healthcare system.

According to a 2020 report from the *National Council of State Boards of Nursing*, accredited programs had a 10% higher NCLEX pass rate than non-accredited programs, emphasizing the link between accreditation and student success. Additionally, accredited programs report higher job placement rates, with 93% of graduates from accredited programs securing employment within six months of graduation (NCBSN, 2020).

1.7 Conclusion

Accreditation in nursing education is a vital process that ensures the quality and effectiveness of nursing programs nationwide. Through rigorous self-assessment, site visits, and continuous monitoring, accreditation provides a framework for improvement and accountability in nursing education. For nursing programs, achieving and maintaining accreditation is not just a regulatory requirement but a critical investment in the quality of education and the professional development of students. As healthcare continues to evolve, accreditation will remain integral to ensuring that nursing programs produce skilled, compassionate, and knowledgeable nurses who can meet the challenges of modern healthcare.

Key Terms

1. **Accreditation**
   The process by which a nursing program is evaluated by a recognized accrediting body to ensure it meets established educational standards and quality.
2. **Accrediting Body**

A recognized organization responsible for assessing nursing programs to ensure they meet specific standards. Examples include the Commission on Collegiate Nursing Education (CCNE) and the Accreditation Commission for Education in Nursing (ACEN).

3. **Self-Study**

An internal evaluation conducted by the nursing program, reviewing its operations, strengths, weaknesses, and compliance with accreditation standards.

4. **Site Visit**

A formal visit by external evaluators from an accrediting body to observe a nursing program's facilities, faculty, and overall operations as part of the accreditation review process.

5. **Continuous Improvement**

The ongoing effort of a nursing program to assess and improve its quality in response to feedback from students, faculty, and external evaluators ensures the program remains current and effective.

6. **Standards of Accreditation**

The criteria set by accrediting bodies that nursing programs must meet include curriculum, faculty qualifications, student outcomes, and resources.

7. **Regional Accreditation**

A form of accreditation that applies to an entire institution, assessing its overall quality. This is separate from programmatic accreditation, which focuses on individual programs like nursing.

8. **Programmatic Accreditation**

Accreditation focusing on individual academic programs, such as nursing, ensures they meet the discipline-specific standards required for high-quality education.

9. **Federal Funding Eligibility**

The requirement for nursing programs to be accredited is to receive federal financial aid and grants for students.

10. **Re-accreditation**

The process by which an accredited nursing program undergoes a review after a set period (typically 3-5 years) to ensure it continues to meet the required standards.

11. **Curriculum Design**

The structure and content of the nursing program's coursework, clinical placements, and overall educational framework must align with accreditation standards.

12. **Student Outcomes**

Measures of success for nursing programs, including graduation rates, licensure exam pass rates, and job placement rates, all of which are evaluated during the accreditation process.

13. **Probationary Status**

A temporary accreditation status is given to a nursing program that fails to meet specific accreditation standards, requiring the program to correct deficiencies before full accreditation is restored.

14. **Faculty Qualifications**

The education, experience, and professional credentials required of instructors in a nursing program are assessed during the accreditation process to ensure faculty meet the standards for effective teaching.

End of Chapter Questions

1. **What is the primary purpose of accreditation for nursing programs?**
   a) To improve faculty salaries

b) To ensure that the program meets established standards for quality and effectiveness

c) To increase the program's enrollment

d) To reduce tuition costs

2. **Which of the following is a primary accrediting body for nursing programs in the United States?**

a) National Institutes of Health (NIH)

b) Commission on Collegiate Nursing Education (CCNE)

c) American Nurses Association (ANA)

d) U.S. Department of Health and Human Services (HHS)

3. **What is the difference between regional and programmatic accreditation in nursing education?**

a) Regional accreditation focuses on specific nursing specialties, while programmatic accreditation evaluates the general curriculum.

b) The federal government requires regional accreditation, while programmatic accreditation is optional.

c) Regional accreditation evaluates the overall institution, while programmatic accreditation evaluates the nursing program specifically.

d) Programmatic accreditation is focused solely on clinical experiences, while regional accreditation focuses on administrative processes.

4. **Which of the following is a benefit of maintaining accreditation for a nursing program?**

a) Increased tuition fees

b) Eligibility for federal funding and grants

c) More lenient faculty hiring requirements

d) Reduced student admission requirements

5. **In the accreditation process, what does a "self-study" involve?**

a) An external review of the program's performance

b) A comprehensive internal assessment of the program's compliance with accreditation standards

c) A written report from the accrediting body regarding their findings

d) A review of faculty credentials only

6. **Why is it essential for a nursing program to demonstrate continuous improvement during the accreditation process?**

a) To avoid financial penalties from the accrediting body

b) To ensure that the program remains relevant, effective, and aligned with evolving healthcare needs

c) To secure more funding from the accrediting agency

d) To prove the nursing program is better than other schools

7. **Which of the following is a common challenge nursing programs face during accreditation?**

a) Lack of student enrollment

b) Insufficient clinical placement opportunities for students

c) Difficulty in meeting accreditation standards related to curriculum design and faculty qualifications

d) Reducing faculty turnover rates

8. **How often do nursing programs typically undergo re-accreditation?**

a) Every year

b) Every 3 to 5 years

c) Every 10 years

d) Only once during the program's lifetime

9. **What is the role of stakeholders (e.g., faculty, students, clinical partners) in the accreditation process?**
   a) They are only consulted once the program has been accredited.
   b) They play a key role in ensuring the program aligns with standards and contributing to the self-study and improvement initiatives.
   c) They are responsible for submitting the application for accreditation.
   d) They are only involved in decision-making regarding faculty salaries.

10. **What is the most common reason a nursing program might not receive initial accreditation?**
   a) Lack of student enrollment
   b) Inability to demonstrate compliance with accreditation standards, such as faculty qualifications or curriculum rigor
   c) The program's focus on research rather than clinical education
   d) Insufficient faculty members employed in the program

Fill in the Blank Questions

1. The primary purpose of accreditation for nursing programs is to ensure that the program meets _____ and _____ standards of quality and effectiveness.
2. The accrediting body responsible for evaluating nursing programs at the baccalaureate and graduate levels is the _____ (CCNE).
3. _____ accreditation evaluates the overall institution, while _____ accreditation evaluates the specific nursing program.
4. One of the benefits of accreditation for nursing programs is eligibility for _____ funding and grants.
5. The accreditation process typically begins with the preparation of a _____, which is an internal assessment of the program's compliance with accreditation standards.
6. During the accreditation process, a key component is the _____ visit, where external reviewers observe the program's operations and verify the information presented in the self-study.
7. Nursing programs must demonstrate _____ improvement to ensure they remain aligned with healthcare industry needs and educational standards.
8. The accreditation body evaluates the program based on criteria such as curriculum design, faculty qualifications, and _____ outcomes.
9. Nursing programs typically undergo re-accreditation every _____ to _____ years.
10. Failure to meet accreditation standards, such as those related to faculty qualifications or clinical placement opportunities, could result in a _____ accreditation status.

Chapter 2
Preparing for Accreditation:
Initial Steps

Accreditation is a cornerstone of quality assurance in nursing education, signifying that a program meets established standards of excellence. For institutions aiming to provide a robust nursing education, the preparation process is both a challenge and an opportunity for growth. By engaging in rigorous self-assessment and aligning with accreditation standards, programs can enhance their reputation, improve student outcomes, and fulfill their mission of preparing competent nursing professionals.

This chapter delves into the initial steps required to set a strong foundation for accreditation. These steps are not simply procedural; they represent a strategic process that reflects an institution's commitment to excellence. From selecting the right accrediting body to forming a capable team, every detail plays a pivotal role in achieving success.

2.1 Identifying the Appropriate Accrediting Body

Choosing the right accrediting body is one of the most fundamental steps in preparing for accreditation, as it sets the tone and direction for the entire process. The accreditor's mission, scope, and evaluation criteria must align with the nursing program's goals, structure, and target audience. This alignment ensures that the accreditation process supports the institution's strategic vision and contributes to meaningful improvements in educational quality.

Overview of Accrediting Bodies

In the United States, nursing programs primarily seek accreditation from the *Accreditation Commission for Education in Nursing* (ACEN) or the *Commission on Collegiate Nursing Education* (CCNE). Both accrediting bodies are recognized by the U.S. Department of Education and the Council for Higher Education Accreditation, ensuring their standards are rigorous and widely respected. However, they differ in focus and applicability:

- **ACEN**: Established in 1938, ACEN accredits many nursing programs, from practical nursing diplomas to doctoral degrees. It emphasizes program outcomes, community engagement, and accessibility, making it suitable for institutions serving diverse populations, including community colleges and technical schools.

- **CCNE**: Founded in 1996, CCNE focuses exclusively on baccalaureate and higher-degree nursing programs. Its standards emphasize leadership, evidence-based practice, and advanced clinical preparation. CCNE accreditation is often associated with programs that develop nursing leaders and advanced practitioners.

In 2022, ACEN accredited approximately 1,200 programs across the United States, while CCNE accredited around 900. Both organizations have shown steady growth in demand, reflecting an increased emphasis on quality assurance in nursing education.

Factors to Consider When Selecting an Accrediting Body

1. Program Type and Level:

The most straightforward consideration is the level of nursing education the institution offers. For example, an Associate Degree in Nursing (ADN) program seeking initial accreditation may find ACEN the best fit due to its extensive experience with associate-level programs. Conversely, a Master of Science in Nursing (MSN) program focusing on advanced clinical and leadership training might benefit more from CCNE accreditation.

2. Institutional Mission and Goals:

An accreditor's philosophy should align with the institution's mission. For instance, a nursing program focused on serving underserved communities might resonate more with ACEN's emphasis on community impact and accessibility. Meanwhile, programs with a research-intensive or leadership-driven mission might find greater synergy with CCNE.

3. Employer and Stakeholder Expectations:

Accreditation also serves as a signal to potential employers, graduate schools, and clinical partners. Some healthcare organizations or state boards of nursing may prefer or even require a specific type of accreditation. For instance, a 2021 survey of healthcare employers revealed that 75% preferred hiring graduates from CCNE-accredited programs for leadership roles, while ACEN-accredited programs were widely recognized for entry-level positions.

4. Geographic Considerations:

One accrediting body may have a stronger presence or historical preference in some states. Understanding regional trends can provide additional insight into which accreditor might be more relevant. For example, ACEN has a robust presence in community and technical colleges in the southeastern United States. At the same time, CCNE dominates in large public universities and private institutions.

Case Study:
Choosing the Right Accreditor

A community college in the Midwest offering an ADN program faced a dilemma when deciding on its accreditor. After evaluating its goals, the college prioritized increasing accessibility and demonstrating its commitment to the local healthcare workforce. Recognizing ACEN's reputation for supporting associate-level programs and its emphasis on outcomes like community engagement and student success, the institution opted for ACEN. Within two years, the college achieved accreditation. It improved its NCLEX pass rate from 78% to 90%, attributing the success to the clear guidance provided by ACEN standards.

Conversely, a large university on the West Coast with a thriving BSN program and an emerging MSN program sought to establish itself as a leader in advanced nursing education. Given its focus on leadership, research, and policy, the university chose CCNE accreditation. By aligning its goals with CCNE's standards, the university enhanced its graduate program enrollment by 35% and secured partnerships with renowned healthcare organizations.

Benefits of Aligning with the Right Accreditor

Programs that select an accreditor aligned with their mission and structure report smoother accreditation processes and better outcomes. According to the National League for Nursing's 2021 survey:

- 85% of programs with a clear accreditor fit completed the process within the expected timeframe.
- 92% reported that the accreditation process enhanced their program's visibility and stakeholder trust.
- Programs experienced an average 15% increase in student enrollment within two years of accreditation.

The Risks of Misalignment

Failure to carefully evaluate accrediting bodies can lead to wasted resources, unmet expectations, or even denial of accreditation. For instance, a nursing program that misjudges the rigor of a chosen accreditor might struggle to meet standards, resulting in costly delays. Programs must ensure their selected accreditor's standards and evaluation processes align with their capacity and goals.

By thoroughly researching accrediting bodies and carefully assessing their alignment with program needs, institutions set the stage for a successful accreditation journey. This initial step facilitates a smoother process and ensures the program's accreditation strengthens its long-term mission and vision.

2.2 Understanding the Accreditation Process: Self-Study, Site Visits, and Review

Once the accrediting body is selected, understanding its accreditation process is critical to a program's success. Accreditation is not a one-time event but a rigorous, multi-phase process that demands meticulous planning, collaboration, and self-reflection. The primary stages—self-study, site visits, and external review—are designed to assess a program's adherence to established standards and its capacity to deliver quality nursing education.

The Accreditation Process: An Overview

Each accrediting body outlines a systematic process for programs to achieve accreditation. While the specific steps may vary, the process typically includes:

1. **Application and Eligibility Determination:** The program submits a formal application and demonstrates that it meets the basic eligibility criteria set by the accreditor, such as offering a curriculum aligned with nursing competencies and having qualified faculty.
2. **Self-Study:** The institution conducts an in-depth self-evaluation, documenting how it meets each standard outlined by the accreditor. This phase is central to the accreditation process.
3. **Site Visit:** External evaluators visit the institution to validate the self-study findings, interview stakeholders, and assess the program's operations.
4. **Accreditation Decision:** The accrediting body reviews all materials, including the self-study report and site visit findings, before deciding on accreditation status.

Self-Study: The Foundation of Accreditation

The self-study is the cornerstone of the accreditation process, requiring programs to critically evaluate their strengths, weaknesses, and opportunities for improvement. It involves comprehensive documentation of how the program meets the accreditor's standards, often across areas such as curriculum design, student outcomes, faculty qualifications, resources, and governance.

1. Developing the Self-Study Report:

Creating a self-study report is a collaborative and resource-intensive process. Programs must gather data, engage stakeholders, and craft evidence-supported narratives. For instance, a nursing program might document its NCLEX-RN pass rates over five years, highlighting trends and interventions taken to improve outcomes. Similarly, faculty credentials, student satisfaction surveys, and clinical partnership agreements must be meticulously compiled.

2. Data Analysis and Continuous Improvement:

The self-study encourages programs to go beyond compliance and focus on continuous quality improvement. For example, suppose a program's attrition rate is higher than desired. In that case, the self-study should outline corrective measures, such as enhanced academic support or mentoring initiatives.

3. Common Challenges in Self-Study Preparation:

Programs often face challenges during the self-study phase, including:

- **Resource Allocation:** Smaller programs may struggle to allocate staff time and financial resources to prepare a robust report.
- **Stakeholder Engagement:** Ensuring active participation from faculty, administrators, students, and external partners can be difficult but is essential for a comprehensive evaluation.
- **Data Gaps:** Missing or incomplete data, such as outdated clinical agreements or missing employment outcomes, can delay the process.

A 2021 *Accreditation Commission for Education in Nursing* (ACEN) survey found that 62% of programs identified self-study as the most challenging accreditation phase, primarily due to the extensive data collection and analysis required.

Site Visits: Validating Compliance and Excellence

Site visits are critical to the accreditation process, allowing external evaluators to observe the program. Typically conducted over two to three days, the site visit is both evaluative and collaborative, allowing accreditors to verify self-study findings and offer guidance.

1. Preparing for the Visit:

Preparation for a site visit begins well before the evaluators arrive. Programs must ensure that documentation is readily accessible, facilities are in optimal condition, and stakeholders are briefed on their roles. Mock site visits, where internal staff or external consultants simulate the accreditor's visit, are increasingly common and help identify potential issues.

2. What Evaluators Look For:

During the visit, accreditors assess multiple facets of the program, including:

- **Curriculum Alignment:** Ensuring that courses meet national nursing competencies and prepare students for licensure.
- **Clinical Experiences:** Evaluating the adequacy and quality of clinical placements, partnerships, and preceptor involvement.
- **Stakeholder Engagement:** Conducting interviews with faculty, students, alumni, and clinical partners to gauge their experiences and perspectives.

For example, a CCNE evaluation team might review clinical logs, observe simulation labs in use, and interview clinical site supervisors to assess whether students are gaining appropriate hands-on experience.

3. The Role of Feedback:

Accreditors provide immediate feedback during the site visit, outlining strengths and areas for improvement. While this feedback is non-binding, programs can address minor issues before the formal review.

External Review and Accreditation Decision

After the site visit, the accreditor's decision-making body reviews all submitted materials and determines the program's accreditation status. Possible outcomes include:

- **Full Accreditation:** Granted for up to 10 years for programs that meet or exceed all standards.
- **Conditional Accreditation:** Issued when deficiencies are identified, requiring the program to address specific areas within a set timeframe.
- **Denial of Accreditation:** Reserved for programs that fail to meet critical standards, often necessitating significant restructuring before reapplication.

In 2022, ACEN reported that 85% of programs achieved full accreditation on their first attempt, 12% received conditional accreditation, and 3% were denied. Common reasons for conditional or denied accreditation included insufficient clinical resources, low licensure exam pass rates, and inadequate faculty qualifications.

2.3 Best Practices for Navigating the Accreditation Process

1. **Start Early:** Programs should prepare at least 18–24 months before their desired accreditation date. Early preparation allows ample time for data collection, stakeholder engagement, and addressing identified gaps.

> **Best Practice**
>
> ➢ Start Early
> ➢ Leverage External Expertise
> ➢ Engage Faculty and Staff
> ➢ Focus on Continuous Improvement

2. **Leverage External Expertise:** Many programs hire accreditation consultants or participate in workshops offered by accrediting bodies to gain insights and guidance.
3. **Engage Faculty and Staff:** Accreditation is a team effort. Faculty and staff involvement strengthens the process and ensures the sustainability of improvements post-accreditation.
4. **Focus on Continuous Improvement:** Rather than treating accreditation as a compliance exercise, programs should use the process to enhance overall quality.

Case Study:

A Community College's Journey to Accreditation

A community college in Texas offering an Associate Degree in Nursing (ADN) program faced challenges during its first attempt at accreditation. Despite having strong NCLEX pass rates (88%), the program lacked formalized policies for clinical site evaluations and struggled with faculty turnover. Recognizing these gaps, the college formed a dedicated accreditation task force and implemented the following changes:

Developed a Comprehensive Clinical Handbook:

This resource outlined evaluation criteria for clinical sites and preceptors, ensuring consistency and compliance.

Invested in Faculty Retention:

Faculty turnover decreased by 40% within a year by offering competitive salaries and professional development opportunities.

When the program reapplied, it achieved full ACEN accreditation, with accreditors praising its robust clinical partnerships and faculty support initiatives.

Understanding and navigating the accreditation process requires diligence, collaboration, and a commitment to excellence. By mastering the self-study phases, site visits, and external reviews, nursing programs can build a strong foundation for achieving and maintaining accreditation.

2.4 Creating an Internal Team: Selecting Key Stakeholders and Staff Members

Establishing an internal accreditation team is a vital early step in the accreditation process. This team serves as the backbone of the institution's efforts, managing the intricacies of the process, ensuring compliance with standards, and fostering collaboration among stakeholders. A well-structured team with diverse expertise can distinguish between a smooth accreditation journey and one fraught with challenges.

Why an Internal Team Matters

Accreditation is a multifaceted process involving comprehensive self-assessment, data analysis, documentation, and stakeholder engagement. Delegating these tasks to a well-chosen team ensures efficiency and accountability. The *Accreditation Commission for Education in Nursing* (ACEN) emphasizes that programs with clearly defined accreditation teams often demonstrate stronger performance in their reviews, as roles and responsibilities are delineated.

A 2021 study by the *National League for Nursing* (NLN) found that institutions with dedicated accreditation committees reduced preparation time by an average of 25% compared to those relying on ad hoc arrangements. This highlights the importance of assembling a cohesive team early in the process.

Core Roles in the Accreditation Team

The makeup of the accreditation team varies based on the size and structure of the nursing program. Still, it typically includes individuals with expertise in administration, academics, data management, and student services. Key roles include:

1. **Accreditation Liaison or Coordinator**

   The cornerstone of the team, this individual manages the accreditation process, serving as the primary point of contact with the accrediting body. They oversee deadlines, organize meetings, and ensure all materials meet required standards. Effective coordinators possess strong organizational skills, attention to detail, and knowledge of accreditation requirements.

   Example: A coordinator at a nursing program undergoing CCNE accreditation maintained a detailed project management system to track progress across all standards, ensuring timely submission of the self-study report.

2. **Faculty Representatives**

   Faculty members play a critical role in accreditation as they directly shape the curriculum, learning outcomes, and teaching practices. Including faculty, representatives ensures that academic standards align with accreditation criteria and fosters a culture of accountability within the faculty team.

3. **Administrative Leaders**

   Leaders such as deans, department chairs, or directors provide strategic oversight, allocate resources, and advocate for the program within the institution. Their involvement is essential for securing funding and institutional support for accreditation initiatives.

4. **Student and Alumni Representatives**

   Including students and alumni in the team can provide valuable perspectives on the program's strengths and weaknesses. For example, alumni feedback on clinical placements or licensure preparation can guide improvements that align with accreditation standards.

5. **Data Specialists and Assessment Experts**

Accreditation relies heavily on data, including metrics like NCLEX pass rates, graduation rates, and employment outcomes. A dedicated data specialist ensures that data collection and analysis are accurate and comprehensive, supporting the self-study and site visit phases.

6. **Clinical Partnership Liaison**

For programs with extensive clinical components, a liaison who manages relationships with clinical sites ensures that these partnerships meet accreditation standards. This role is especially critical for demonstrating compliance with criteria related to hands-on training.

7. **Support Staff**

The support staff will provide information throughout the process, including helping collect data, cleaning data up, reviewing current processes, and providing expertise in their areas (e.g., student affairs, clinical placement, compliance, simulation)

Accreditation Coordinator	Faculty
Administrative Leader(s)	Student/Alumni Reps
Data Specialist	Clinical Partnership Liaison
Support Staff	

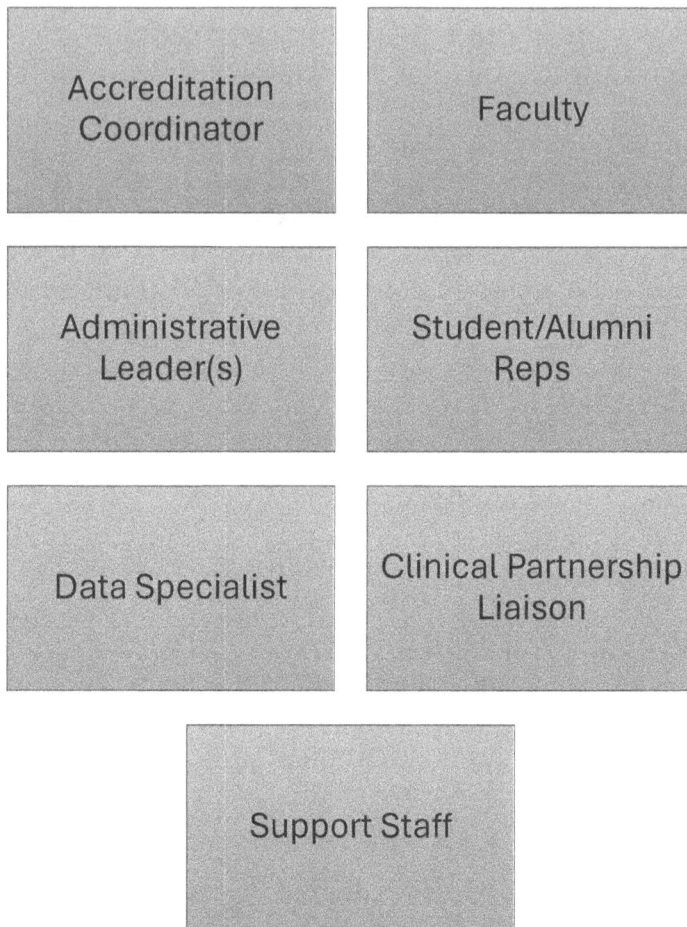

Figure 4 Core Roles for the Accreditation Team

Building the Team: Selection Criteria

When forming the team, programs must carefully select qualified and committed individuals for the accreditation process. Key selection criteria include:

- **Experience and Expertise:** Members should have a strong understanding of their respective areas, such as curriculum design, assessment, or student services.

- **Collaborative Skills:** Accreditation requires teamwork and open communication. Select individuals who can work effectively with others and contribute to a positive team dynamic.
- **Commitment to Quality:** Members must view accreditation as an opportunity for continuous improvement rather than a compliance exercise.

Challenges in Team Formation

Building an effective accreditation team is not without its challenges. Common obstacles include:

1. **Time Constraints:** Faculty and staff often juggle accreditation responsibilities with their regular duties, leading to burnout or conflicts in prioritization.
2. **Resource Limitations:** Smaller programs may lack the personnel to dedicate individuals solely to the accreditation process.
3. **Resistance to Change:** Team members who view accreditation as an unnecessary burden may hinder progress, requiring strategic leadership to foster a shared sense of purpose.

Best Practices for Team Success

1. **Provide Training:** Accrediting bodies often offer workshops, webinars, and resources to familiarize teams with the accreditation process. Institutions should invest in this training to build capacity and confidence.
2. **Define Roles Clearly:** Establishing clear responsibilities for each team member reduces overlap and ensures accountability.
3. **Maintain Regular Communication:** Weekly or biweekly meetings align the team, address emerging challenges, and maintain momentum.
4. **Celebrate Milestones:** Recognizing achievements, such as completing the self-study draft or submitting required documents, boosts morale and reinforces the team's commitment.

Case Study:

Building an Effective Team

A small rural college in the Midwest preparing for its first ACEN accreditation faced challenges due to limited staffing. To overcome this, the dean formed a cross-functional team that included faculty, administrative staff, and clinical site managers. Recognizing the need for data expertise, the college hired a part-time consultant to assist with analytics and reporting.

The team adopted project management software to foster collaboration, enabling real-time updates and task tracking. They also held monthly progress reviews and celebrated small successes, such as meeting NCLEX pass rate benchmarks. The team had prepared a thorough self-study report by the time of the site visit. It strengthened the program's internal communication and processes.

The Long-Term Impact of a Strong Team

Beyond accreditation, the internal team's work often leaves a lasting impact on the program. By fostering a continuous improvement and collaboration culture, the team's efforts can set the stage for sustained excellence. Programs that successfully navigate accreditation often report increased faculty engagement, improved student outcomes, and enhanced institutional reputation.

Creating an effective internal team is essential in the accreditation journey. With the right mix of expertise, collaboration, and commitment, the team becomes the driving force behind a program's success in achieving and maintaining accreditation.

2.5 Developing a Timeline and Action Plan for Accreditation Preparation

Accreditation is a meticulous process that demands careful planning, organization, and adherence to deadlines. Developing a comprehensive timeline and action plan is critical to ensuring that every aspect of the accreditation process is addressed systematically. A detailed plan keeps the accreditation team on track and helps the program manage resources effectively and meet key milestones.

The Importance of a Timeline and Action Plan

An accreditation timeline provides a clear roadmap for the preparation process, helping to prevent last-minute scrambles and overlooked requirements. Accrediting bodies such as the *Commission on Collegiate Nursing Education* (CCNE) and the *Accreditation Commission for Education in Nursing* (ACEN) often publish specific timelines for submission of self-study reports, site visits, and final decisions. Adhering to these deadlines is essential, as missing them can result in costly delays or, in some cases, a denial of accreditation.

A 2019 study published in *Nursing Education Perspectives* revealed that nursing programs with well-defined action plans completed their accreditation preparations 30% faster than those without, underscoring the value of early and effective planning.

Key Steps in Developing a Timeline

1. **Understand the Accreditation Process and Requirements**

   The first step in creating a timeline is thoroughly understanding the accrediting body's requirements. This includes familiarizing the team with deadlines for submitting an intent to seek accreditation, self-study reports, and required fees. It also involves reviewing the accreditor's handbook or guidelines to identify major milestones.

   Example: The ACEN requires programs to submit a candidacy eligibility application at least one year before the planned site visit. Programs must consider this lead time when establishing their timelines.

2. **Set Realistic Deadlines for Internal Milestones**

   Break down the process into manageable phases, such as conducting a self-assessment, drafting the self-study report, and preparing for the site visit. Assign deadlines to each phase based on the accreditor's overall timeline, allowing some buffer time to address unexpected challenges.

3. **Engage Stakeholders in Timeline Development**

   Collaborating with faculty, administrators, and other team members ensures the timeline is realistic and accounts for existing workload constraints. Input from stakeholders also fosters buy-in and accountability.

4. **Incorporate Regular Checkpoints**

   Include regular progress reviews to ensure the team remains on track. These checkpoints allow for early identification of delays or obstacles, enabling timely course corrections.

Creating an Action Plan

An action plan complements the timeline by detailing the tasks required to achieve each milestone. It assigns responsibility to team members, outlines resource needs, and establishes performance indicators to measure progress. Key components of an effective action plan include:

1. **Task Allocation**

Assign tasks to specific team members based on their expertise. For example, data specialists may handle NCLEX pass rate analysis. At the same time, faculty members may focus on aligning the curriculum with accreditation standards.

2. **Resource Allocation**

Accreditation preparation often requires additional resources, such as funding for workshops, technology upgrades, or hiring consultants. The action plan should outline these resource needs and identify sources of funding or support.

3. **Contingency Planning**

Anticipate potential challenges, such as staff turnover, data collection issues, or delays in approval processes. Develop contingency plans to address these risks without derailing the overall timeline.

4. **Monitoring and Reporting**

Establish mechanisms for tracking progress and reporting it to institutional leaders. Regular updates ensure accountability and maintain focus on achieving accreditation goals.

Best Practices for Timelines and Action Plans

1. **Start Early:** Accreditation preparation often takes 18–24 months. Starting early provides ample time to address deficiencies or gaps identified during the self-assessment phase.
2. **Use Project Management Tools:** Tools like Gantt charts, Trello, or Microsoft Project can help visualize the timeline, track tasks, and coordinate team efforts.
3. **Align with Academic Calendars:** Coordinate accreditation activities with the academic calendar to minimize disruptions, such as avoiding critical deadlines during peak teaching periods or holidays.
4. **Seek Feedback:** Periodically review the timeline and action plan with external consultants or accrediting body representatives to ensure alignment with expectations.

Challenges in Timeline Development

1. **Unrealistic Deadlines:** Overly ambitious timelines can lead to burnout among team members and rushed work that may not meet accreditation standards.
2. **Insufficient Buy-In:** Resistance from faculty or staff can impede progress, particularly if they feel excluded from the planning process.
3. **Unanticipated Delays:** External factors, such as changes in accreditation standards or administrative turnover, can disrupt even the best-laid plans.

Case Example:

Streamlining the Accreditation Process

A mid-sized nursing program in California used a detailed timeline and action plan to achieve CCNE accreditation. The program began by forming a task force and conducting a comprehensive gap analysis. Based on the analysis, they created a two-year timeline that included:

Phase 1: Initial preparation, including selecting team members, gathering baseline data, and attending an accreditation workshop.

Phase 2: Conducting a self-assessment and drafting the self-study report over nine months.

Phase 3: Preparing for the site visit, including training staff and conducting mock site reviews.

To manage progress, the program used a project management platform to assign tasks, set deadlines, and monitor completion rates. Despite facing unexpected challenges, such as a faculty turnover rate of 15% during the preparation phase, the team completed their accreditation on time, receiving full approval with commendations for their self-study organization.

Impact of a Robust Timeline and Plan

Developing a detailed timeline and action plan benefits the accreditation process and the program's operations. The process often highlights inefficiencies, such as outdated data management practices or communication gaps, prompting broader improvements. For instance, a 2022 *American Association of Colleges of Nursing* (AACN) survey found that 78% of nursing programs that achieved accreditation reported enhanced internal processes as a byproduct of their preparation efforts.

In conclusion, a well-constructed timeline and action plan are essential for navigating the complex accreditation process. They provide structure, promote accountability, and ensure that all required tasks are completed on schedule. Nursing programs can approach accreditation with confidence and clarity by following best practices and engaging stakeholders.

2.6 Assessing the Program's Current State: Strengths and Areas for Improvement

Before embarking on the accreditation journey, nursing programs must thoroughly and honestly evaluate their current state. This assessment is the foundation for identifying strengths that align with accreditation standards and uncovering areas that need improvement. Accrediting bodies such as the *Accreditation Commission for Education in Nursing* (ACEN) and the *Commission on Collegiate Nursing Education* (CCNE) emphasize the importance of self-assessment in achieving accreditation readiness.

The Role of Self-Assessment in Accreditation

Self-assessment is a structured process that involves evaluating the program's policies, practices, outcomes, and alignment with accreditation criteria. This step is essential for uncovering discrepancies between current practices and the standards set forth by accrediting agencies. A comprehensive self-assessment clarifies the program's readiness for accreditation and provides a roadmap for improvements that will enhance the program's quality and sustainability.

A 2021 report by the *American Association of Colleges of Nursing* (AACN) found that nursing programs that conducted detailed self-assessments were 25% more likely to achieve initial accreditation on their first attempt than programs that overlooked this step.

Steps in Assessing the Program

1. **Review Accreditation Standards**

   Begin by familiarizing the accreditation team with the accrediting body's standards and criteria. These standards often include curriculum quality, student learning outcomes, faculty qualifications, resource adequacy, and institutional support.

   Example: CCNE accreditation standards require programs to demonstrate compliance in four primary areas: mission and governance, institutional commitment, curriculum and teaching-learning practices, and program effectiveness.

2. **Gather and Analyze Data**

Data collection is central to the self-assessment process. Programs must gather quantitative and qualitative data that reflect their current state. Key data points may include:

- o **Student Outcomes:** Graduation rates, NCLEX pass rates, job placement rates, and student satisfaction scores.
- o **Faculty Qualifications:** Percentage of faculty with terminal degrees, teaching experience, and engagement in professional development.
- o **Resource Metrics:** Availability of clinical sites, technology, library resources, and simulation labs.
- o **Curriculum Alignment:** How well the curriculum meets current professional and regulatory requirements.

For instance, the *National Council of State Boards of Nursing* (NCSBN) reported that in 2022 the national average first-time NCLEX pass rate was 79%. A program with a lower pass rate may identify this as a priority area for improvement.

3. **Conduct Stakeholder Surveys and Focus Groups**

Gathering input from stakeholders, including students, faculty, alumni, and employers, provides a well-rounded view of the program's strengths and weaknesses. Stakeholder feedback can reveal gaps not immediately evident from quantitative data alone.

Example: Surveys of recent graduates might reveal dissatisfaction with clinical placement opportunities, prompting the program to strengthen partnerships with healthcare facilities.

4. **Evaluate Compliance with Accreditation Standards**

Use a rubric or checklist to evaluate the program's performance against each accreditation criterion. For example, if an accrediting body requires evidence of continuous quality improvement (CQI), assess whether the program has established mechanisms for monitoring and enhancing quality.

5. **Identify Gaps and Prioritize Improvements**

Based on the data analysis and evaluation, identify specific gaps that must be addressed. Prioritize these gaps based on their potential impact on the accreditation process and the program's overall quality.

Example: Low faculty retention rates may signal a need for enhanced professional development or workload adjustments to retain qualified instructors.

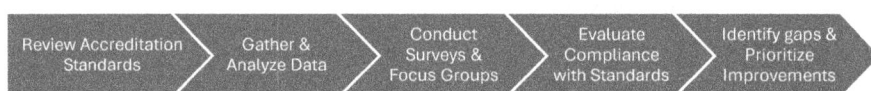

Figure 5 Pre-Self-study: Assessing Your Program

Common Areas of Strength

- **High NCLEX Pass Rates:** Programs consistently exceeding national averages demonstrate strong curriculum design and effective teaching methods.
- **Qualified Faculty:** Faculty with advanced degrees and active involvement in research or professional organizations often contribute to a program's credibility.
- **Innovative Curriculum:** Programs incorporating emerging trends, such as telehealth training or interprofessional education, may stand out as leaders in nursing education.

Common Areas for Improvement

1. **Curriculum Gaps:** Many programs struggle with aligning their curriculum with evolving healthcare demands. For example, a lack of content on culturally competent care or health informatics may be identified as a gap.
2. **Insufficient Resources:** Limited access to clinical sites, outdated simulation equipment, or inadequate library resources can hinder student learning and program effectiveness.

3. **Data Collection and Analysis:** Programs often lack robust systems for tracking and analyzing key performance metrics, such as graduate outcomes or employer satisfaction.
4. **Faculty Turnover:** High turnover rates can disrupt continuity and negatively impact student outcomes. A 2020 AACN report found that faculty shortages affected 48% of nursing programs in the U.S., limiting their ability to maintain quality standards.

Case Study:

Assessing the State of a Rural Nursing Program

A rural nursing program preparing for ACEN accreditation conducted a detailed self-assessment. Key findings included:

Strengths:
- NCLEX pass rates of 85%, exceeding national averages.
- A dedicated faculty team with 90% holding master's degrees.
- Strong partnerships with local healthcare providers for clinical placements.

Areas for Improvement:
- Limited simulation lab capacity, leading to scheduling conflicts.
- Curriculum lacked dedicated coursework on telehealth and geriatric care.
- Faculty retention challenges due to competitive salaries in urban areas.

Based on these findings, the program prioritized upgrading its simulation lab and revising its curriculum to address gaps. These changes enhanced the program's quality and positioned it for a successful accreditation outcome.

Benefits of a Comprehensive Assessment

1. **Clarity and Focus:** Self-assessment clarifies what the program is doing well and where it needs to improve, enabling focused efforts and efficient resource allocation.
2. **Improved Stakeholder Engagement:** Involving faculty, students, and administrators in the assessment process fosters a sense of ownership and commitment to the program's goals.
3. **Strengthened Strategic Planning:** The insights gained from self-assessment inform long-term planning, ensuring the program remains responsive to changes in the healthcare and education landscape.

Assessing the current state of a nursing program is a cornerstone of the accreditation preparation process. By systematically evaluating strengths and areas for improvement, programs can align their efforts with accreditation standards and enhance their overall quality. This step ensures a smoother accreditation process and supports the long-term success of the program, its students, and the healthcare community it serves.

2.7 Setting Goals and Objectives for Achieving Accreditation

Once a nursing program has thoroughly assessed its current state, the next crucial step is setting clear, achievable goals and objectives to guide its path toward accreditation. This process provides the program with a structured framework for improvement. It ensures that all efforts are aligned with the accreditation standards. Setting specific goals helps create a sense of purpose, fosters stakeholder collaboration, and provides measurable benchmarks to track progress.

Why Goal Setting is Critical for Accreditation Success

Goal setting is fundamental because it transforms abstract ideas into actionable plans. By breaking down the accreditation process into manageable objectives, nursing programs can prioritize improvements, allocate resources efficiently, and monitor progress effectively. Furthermore, well-defined goals ensure that the program remains focused on the accreditation standards and avoids becoming distracted by unrelated issues.

A study published in the *Journal of Nursing Education and Practice* found that nursing programs that implemented a structured goal-setting process saw a 30% higher success rate in achieving accreditation than those that did not. This demonstrates how the strategic alignment of goals with accreditation criteria directly influences a program's ability to meet and secure accreditation standards.

SMART Goals: A Framework for Success

To ensure that goals are achievable and measurable, many nursing programs adopt the SMART criteria—an acronym for Specific, Measurable, Achievable, Relevant, and Time-bound. This framework helps ensure that goals are clear and trackable, promoting accountability among all stakeholders involved in the accreditation process.

1. **Specific:**

   The goal should be unambiguous, outlining exactly what needs to be accomplished.

   Example: "Increase NCLEX pass rates by 10% over the next two years."

2. **Measurable:** There should be concrete criteria to track progress and determine when the goal has been met.

   Example: "Enhance student satisfaction with clinical placements, measured by a 15% increase in positive survey responses."

3. **Achievable:** The goal should be realistic, given the program's resources, capabilities, and time constraints.

   Example: "Introduce a faculty development program to improve clinical teaching skills within a year."

4. **Relevant:** The goal should align with the program's mission and contribute to the accreditation standards.

   Example: "Improve faculty retention by offering professional development opportunities, which will directly contribute to meeting accreditation standards related to faculty qualifications."

5. **Time-bound:** There should be a clear timeline for achieving the goal, with deadlines to ensure accountability.

   Example: "Complete a curriculum review and revision process by the end of the upcoming academic year."

By applying the SMART framework, nursing programs can create a structured roadmap that ensures progress toward accreditation while maintaining alignment with long-term objectives.

Setting Program-Specific Goals

A nursing program's goals will depend on its unique challenges, opportunities, and focus areas. However, common goals that many programs may need to set as part of their accreditation preparation include:

1. **Curriculum Enhancement:**

   A well-aligned curriculum is a core component of accreditation. Nursing programs must often revise or enhance their curriculum to meet the latest industry standards and address emerging healthcare needs. For example, a program might set a goal to integrate more content on health information technology, mental health, or geriatric care, depending on the program's areas of weakness.

Example Goal: "Revise the nursing curriculum to incorporate evidence-based practices, focusing on culturally competent care, by the end of the next academic year."

2. Improving Faculty Qualifications and Development:

One of the key accreditation standards is the quality and qualifications of faculty members. Suppose a program identifies gaps in faculty credentials. In that case, it should set goals to improve faculty qualifications through professional development, recruitment, or mentoring.

Example Goal: "Increase the percentage of faculty with doctoral degrees from 60% to 75% over the next three years."

3. Enhancing Student Outcomes

Accreditation agencies require data on student outcomes, including NCLEX pass rates, graduation rates, and employment rates. Programs often set goals to improve these outcomes by strengthening student support services, increasing clinical exposure, and refining teaching methods.

Example Goal: "Increase NCLEX first-time pass rates from 80% to 90% over the next two years by enhancing test preparation resources and clinical practice hours."

4. Strengthening Clinical Partnerships and Resources:

Accreditation bodies emphasize a program's ability to provide adequate clinical training opportunities. If a program is struggling to secure enough clinical sites or has issues with clinical faculty, setting a goal to build stronger partnerships with local hospitals, clinics, and healthcare providers is vital.

Example Goal: "Establish two new clinical partnerships with local hospitals within the next year to ensure 100% of students have access to high-quality clinical placements."

5. Improving Resource Allocation:

Adequate resources, such as faculty, funding, technology, and simulation labs, are essential for nursing programs to meet accreditation standards. Goals in this area may focus on securing additional funding, upgrading equipment, or improving infrastructure to support the program's objectives.

Example Goal: "Increase funding for simulation equipment by 25% within the next fiscal year to support enhanced clinical training opportunities."

6. **Building a Continuous Quality Improvement (CQI) Program:**

Many accreditation bodies require evidence of continuous quality improvement efforts. A program might set a goal to develop or enhance its CQI initiatives by incorporating regular program reviews, gathering stakeholder feedback, and making adjustments based on data-driven decisions.

Example Goal: "Establish a continuous quality improvement program within six months, including quarterly assessments of student outcomes, clinical placements, and faculty performance."

Involving Stakeholders in Goal Setting

Effective goal setting for accreditation is not solely the responsibility of the administration; it requires input from various stakeholders within the nursing program. Engaging faculty, staff, students, and external partners in the goal-setting process ensures that the goals are realistic, relevant, and supported by those responsible for implementing them.

- **Faculty:** Involve faculty members in identifying goals related to curriculum, pedagogy, and student support. Their expertise ensures that goals are educationally sound and aligned with accreditation standards.
- **Students:** Gather input from current and former students to understand their needs and concerns. Their perspectives can help identify areas where the program may need to improve its approach to teaching and student outcomes.
- **Clinical Partners:** Collaborate with clinical partners to identify gaps in clinical training and ensure that goals related to clinical placements and partnerships are feasible.
- **Alumni and Employers:** Alumni and employers offer valuable insights into how well the program prepares graduates for real-world nursing

practice. Their feedback can inform goals related to student outcomes, employability, and program relevance.

Tracking Progress and Adjusting Goals

Once goals are set, tracking progress regularly is important to ensure the program is progressing toward accreditation readiness. Establishing a monitoring system will allow the accreditation team to evaluate whether the goals are being met and adjustments are needed. Programs can use tools such as project management software, dashboards, and regular progress meetings to stay on track.

Example: If a program is not meeting its NCLEX pass rate goals, it may need to adjust its strategies, such as increasing student remediation efforts, improving clinical training, or providing additional test preparation resources.

Setting clear, measurable, and realistic goals is essential for accreditation preparation. By applying the SMART framework and aligning goals with accreditation standards, nursing programs can stay focused on their objectives and ensure that they are making meaningful progress toward accreditation. Involving all stakeholders in this process fosters collaboration. It ensures that the program is positioned to achieve and maintain accreditation, ultimately enhancing the quality of nursing education and healthcare delivery.

2.8 Conclusion

Chapter 2 of this book focuses on the essential steps of nursing programs to prepare for accreditation. It provides an in-depth look at setting up a solid foundation for achieving and maintaining accreditation, beginning with identifying the appropriate accrediting body. The chapter emphasizes understanding the accreditation process, which typically involves conducting a self-study, hosting site visits, and undergoing a comprehensive review by the accrediting agency.

A critical step is assembling an internal team, including key stakeholders and staff members, who will guide and manage the accreditation efforts. This team should be diverse, representing different aspects of the program, including faculty, administration, and clinical partners, to ensure that all program areas are adequately represented and addressed.

The chapter also highlights the importance of developing a detailed timeline and action plan for accreditation preparation. This plan should break down tasks into manageable stages, with clear deadlines to keep the program on track. Integral to this preparation is a thorough assessment of the program's current state, identifying strengths and areas for improvement. This self-assessment serves as a baseline for setting specific, achievable goals.

Finally, the chapter discusses the importance of setting SMART (Specific, Measurable, Achievable, Relevant, and Time-bound) goals for achieving accreditation. These goals should address key areas like curriculum enhancement, faculty development, student outcomes, and clinical partnerships. By involving all stakeholders in the goal-setting process, nursing programs can create a shared vision for accreditation success and ensure that resources are allocated efficiently to meet the standards.

Chapter 2 provides the necessary framework and guidance for nursing programs to begin their accreditation journey. Through careful planning, goal setting, and collaboration, programs can position themselves for success in achieving and maintaining accreditation.

Key Terms for Chapter 2

1. **Accreditation**
    The formal recognition by an authoritative body (e.g., CCNE, ACEN) that a nursing program meets established quality standards in education, operations, and outcomes.

2. **Accrediting Body**
    An organization that evaluates and grants accreditation to nursing programs based on their compliance with established criteria, such as CCNE or ACEN.

3. **Self-Study**
    A comprehensive, reflective process in which a nursing program assesses its operations, strengths, weaknesses, and alignment with accreditation standards. This document is submitted to accrediting bodies.

4. **Site Visit**
    A visit by the accrediting body's evaluation team to assess a nursing program's compliance with accreditation standards. This is typically an on-site review of facilities, curriculum, and outcomes.

5. **Stakeholders**
    Individuals or groups interested in the nursing program's success and accreditation process include faculty, administrators, students, alumni, clinical partners, and governing bodies.

6. **Action Plan**
    A detailed plan that outlines the steps, timeline, and resources needed to address areas of improvement identified during the accreditation preparation process.

7. **Timeline**

A detailed schedule that outlines the specific steps, milestones, and deadlines for completing tasks involved in preparing for accreditation, including the self-study, documentation, and site visit preparation.

8. **Gap Analysis**

The process of evaluating a nursing program's current state in relation to accreditation standards, identifying areas of improvement or non-compliance that need to be addressed before applying for accreditation.

9. **Program Evaluation**

The ongoing assessment of a nursing program's effectiveness, including curriculum, faculty performance, student outcomes, and organizational processes. This is often part of the accreditation self-study process.

10. **Continuous Improvement**

A commitment to ongoing evaluation and enhancement of the nursing program, ensuring that standards are met and exceeded over time. This is integral to maintaining accreditation status.

11. **Accreditation Standards**

Specific criteria and requirements set by the accrediting body that a nursing program must meet to achieve and maintain accreditation. These include faculty qualifications, curriculum quality, clinical experiences, and student outcomes.

12. **Documentation**

The written materials and evidence (such as syllabi, curriculum maps, faculty qualifications, and student outcome data) are required for the accreditation process.

13. **Quality Assurance**

Systematic efforts are made to ensure the nursing program consistently meets high education standards, clinical training, and outcomes. Quality assurance processes are often assessed during accreditation reviews.

14. **Faculty Development**

Training and professional growth opportunities for nursing faculty to improve teaching skills, stay current with nursing trends, and align with accreditation standards.

15. **Resource Allocation**

The process of efficiently distributing resources, such as budget, faculty, and clinical sites, to ensure the nursing program meets the necessary standards for accreditation.

16. **Curriculum Mapping**

The process of aligning the nursing program's curriculum with accreditation standards to ensure that educational objectives are achieved and appropriate content is covered.

17. **Peer Review**

A process where faculty, administrators, and other professionals evaluate a nursing program's strengths and areas for improvement, contributing to the self-study process.

18. **External Review Team**
    A group of experts in nursing education and practice selected by the accrediting body to evaluate the program's compliance with accreditation standards during the site visit.

19. **Program Outcomes**
    Specific, measurable achievements of a nursing program include graduation rates, NCLEX pass rates, and employment rates of graduates. These outcomes are critical components in the accreditation process.

20. **Regulatory Compliance**
    Ensuring that the nursing program adheres to federal, state, and accrediting body regulations, which can include curriculum requirements, faculty qualifications, and student support services

End of Chapter 2 Questions

1. What is the first step a nursing program should take when preparing for accreditation, and why is it important?
2. Describe the key components involved in the accreditation process.
3. Why is forming an internal team when preparing for accreditation important, and who should be included?
4. What are some key factors to consider when creating a timeline for accreditation preparation?
5. How does conducting a gap analysis help a nursing program prepare for accreditation?
6. What common challenges do nursing programs face during accreditation preparation, and how can they be mitigated?
7. Explain the role of program outcomes in the accreditation process and how they contribute to a program's success.
8. What is the purpose of the self-study in the accreditation process, and what should it include?
9. Why is stakeholder engagement critical in the accreditation preparation process, and how can it be effectively achieved?
10. How can nursing programs ensure they meet the expectations of accrediting bodies while maintaining their unique characteristics and strengths?

Fill in the Blank Questions

1. The first step in preparing for accreditation is to identify the appropriate _____ for your nursing program.
2. The accreditation process typically involves conducting a _____, preparing for a _____, and undergoing a _____ by the accrediting body.
3. A nursing program should form an internal team to ensure that all necessary _____ are considered when preparing for accreditation.
4. When creating a timeline for accreditation preparation, it is important to consider the accreditation body's _____, faculty and staff involvement, and sufficient time for documentation.

5. Conducting a _____ helps identify areas where the nursing program does not meet accreditation standards, providing a clear roadmap for improvements.

6. A _____ study is a comprehensive internal assessment that details how a nursing program meets or plans to meet accreditation standards.

7. Nursing programs must demonstrate _____ through program outcomes such as graduation rates, NCLEX pass rates, and employment rates to meet accreditation requirements.

8. Effective _____ engagement is critical during accreditation preparation, as it ensures that all stakeholders, including faculty, students, and clinical partners, are involved in the process.

9. The process of _____ provides a clear plan for addressing any areas of weakness or non-compliance in the nursing program during accreditation preparation.

10. The _____ visit is an on-site evaluation by the accrediting body to assess a nursing program's adherence to accreditation standards.

Chapter 3
Self-Study and Documentation

The self-study process is the cornerstone of any successful accreditation effort, functioning as both a roadmap for program improvement and a comprehensive reflection of a nursing program's quality. This essential phase requires a detailed evaluation of all program components, including mission alignment, curriculum design, student outcomes, and faculty qualifications. Beyond being an exercise in compliance, the self-study allows programs to align their operations with industry standards and strengthen their foundation for long-term success.

The stakes of the self-study process are high. Accrediting bodies rely heavily on this document to evaluate a program's readiness for accreditation. A poorly executed self-study can lead to delays, additional scrutiny, or even denial of accreditation, which can have severe consequences, such as decreased enrollment or funding challenges. Conversely, a well-crafted self-study demonstrates a program's dedication to excellence, often leading to enhanced reputation and more robust stakeholder support.

3.1 Importance of the Self-Study Process in Accreditation

The self-study process is the foundation for achieving accreditation, reflecting a nursing program's current state and a strategic guide for future improvement. At its core, the self-study provides a comprehensive and structured evaluation of every aspect of the program, from curriculum design and faculty qualifications to student outcomes and resource allocation. This document is not merely an exercise in compliance but a critical tool that promotes self-awareness, accountability, and continuous improvement.

The Role of the Self-Study in Accreditation

The self-study document is one of the most critical components accreditation bodies use to assess whether a program meets the established quality standards. It demonstrates the program's commitment to excellence, innovation, and alignment with industry needs. Accrediting organizations such as the *Commission on Collegiate Nursing Education* (CCNE) and the *Accreditation Commission for Education in Nursing* (ACEN) rely heavily on self-study to evaluate a program's readiness for accreditation. Programs that fail to address accreditation criteria through their self-study adequately often face delays or additional scrutiny, which can jeopardize their accreditation status.

Statistics from ACEN show that over 85% of nursing programs receiving full accreditation on their first attempt invested significant time—typically 12 to 18 months—in crafting a robust self-study. This preparation demonstrates the importance of taking the process seriously and dedicating sufficient resources to ensure the document is thorough and accurate.

A Catalyst for Self-Reflection

Beyond satisfying external requirements, the self-study process is a powerful tool for internal reflection. Programs are encouraged to take an honest and critical look at their strengths, weaknesses, and areas for growth. This internal assessment often uncovers issues that might not have been apparent during day-to-day operations. For example, a program might discover during the self-study process that while its NCLEX pass rates are high, its graduation rates are below the national average, potentially indicating a need to reevaluate student support services or curriculum sequencing.

Such insights enhance the program's ability to secure accreditation and position it for long-term success. Programs that actively embrace self-study as a means of self-improvement often find that the benefits extend well beyond the accreditation cycle, leading to better student outcomes, improved faculty satisfaction, and more substantial alignment with community needs.

Benefits of the Self-Study for Stakeholders

The self-study also creates value for the program's various stakeholders. For faculty and staff, the process clarifies institutional goals and fosters collaboration. Faculty members learn how their roles contribute to the program's broader mission. At the same time, staff can better understand how their efforts support student success.

For students, a well-executed self-study translates to a more robust program overall. Accreditation ensures that students receive an education that meets national standards, which is critical for their professional development and employability. In addition, engaging students in the self-study process—through surveys, focus groups, or feedback sessions—helps institutions identify areas where the student experience can be improved.

The self-study demonstrates the program's commitment to accountability and excellence for external stakeholders, such as clinical partners and community organizations. This can strengthen partnerships, open new opportunities for collaboration, and enhance the program's reputation within the healthcare community.

An Investment in the Program's Future

The self-study process is resource-intensive, requiring significant time, personnel, and funding. However, the investment pays off in multiple ways. Programs that approach the process with diligence and intentionality often see tangible benefits, such as increased enrollment, stronger alumni engagement, and enhanced institutional reputation.

One illustrative example comes from a mid-sized nursing program in the Midwest. It used its self-study to identify a gap in its clinical partnerships. The program strengthened its accreditation application by addressing this gap and building new relationships with local healthcare providers. It provided students with more diverse and high-quality clinical experiences. As a result, the program saw a 25% increase in student satisfaction scores and a 15% rise in job placement rates within two years.

Challenges and Consequences of Neglecting the Self-Study

While the self-study offers numerous benefits, it can also present challenges. Programs that fail to allocate adequate time or resources often struggle to meet deadlines or produce documents that satisfy accreditation requirements. This can lead to significant consequences, including probationary accreditation status, reputational damage, and even loss of eligibility to participate in federal financial aid programs.

A 2019 study published in the *Journal of Nursing Education and Practice* found that nursing programs receiving probationary accreditation cited deficiencies in their self-study documents as the most common issue, with 62% reporting incomplete data or poorly articulated outcomes. These findings underscore the importance of meticulous planning and execution during self-study.

The Self-Study as a Continuous Process

Finally, it is essential to view the self-study not as a one-time task but as an ongoing process. Programs should continuously collect data, evaluate their performance, and refine their practices even outside the formal accreditation cycle. This proactive approach simplifies future self-study efforts and ensures that the program remains agile and responsive to changes in the healthcare landscape.

In conclusion, the self-study process is vital in achieving and maintaining accreditation. It requires significant effort and resources, but the immediate and long-term benefits are invaluable. By embracing self-study as a reflection, improvement, and accountability tool, nursing programs can position themselves for success in a competitive and ever-changing educational environment.

3.2 Structuring the Self-Study Document: Key Components

A well-structured self-study document is essential for accreditation success. Accrediting bodies rely on this document to assess whether a nursing program meets the rigorous standards to ensure educational excellence and graduate readiness. Each section of the self-study should be clear, evidence-based, and aligned with the specific criteria the chosen accrediting agency sets forth. A systematic approach to structuring the document ensures that no critical areas are overlooked and that the program presents a coherent narrative of its strengths and areas for improvement.

Mission and Vision Statements

The foundation of the self-study lies in the mission and vision statements. These declarations serve as guiding principles for the nursing program, encapsulating its purpose and aspirations. Accrediting agencies expect these statements to align with the institution's overall mission while reflecting the unique goals of the nursing program.

For instance, the mission statement might focus on preparing graduates to deliver compassionate, evidence-based care in diverse settings. At the same time, the vision could emphasize becoming a regional leader in nursing education. These statements provide a framework for the rest of the self-study, ensuring that all subsequent components tie back to the program's overarching purpose.

Accreditation Standards and Mission Alignment

The accrediting body evaluates how well the program's mission and vision align with its curriculum, resources, and outcomes. For example, if the mission emphasizes community health, the program should demonstrate partnerships with local organizations and evidence of student involvement in community-based clinical experiences. Failure to align the mission and vision with program practices can weaken the self-study's credibility.

Program Outcomes and Goals

Program outcomes and goals form another critical section of the self-study. These metrics define the program's aims and how success is measured. Typical outcomes include NCLEX-RN pass rates, graduation rates, employment rates, and student satisfaction. Goals often encompass objectives related to faculty development, curriculum enhancement, or expanding clinical partnerships.

Evidence of Achievement

Accrediting bodies require programs to provide quantitative and qualitative evidence of achieving these outcomes. For instance, if a program aims to maintain an 85% NCLEX pass rate, it must include historical data demonstrating this achievement. Additionally, the program should outline strategies for addressing gaps, such as enhanced test preparation resources or curriculum adjustments.

Benchmarking Against National Standards

Benchmarking is a key practice in this section. Programs should compare their outcomes to national averages and peer institutions. According to the *National Council of State Boards of Nursing* (NCSBN), the national average first-time NCLEX-RN pass rate for U.S. nursing programs was approximately 79.9% in 2021. Programs exceeding this benchmark can highlight their success, while those below it should provide action plans for improvement.

Faculty Qualifications and Resources

The quality and credentials of the faculty are critical components of the self-study. Accrediting agencies require detailed information about faculty qualifications, including degrees earned, clinical expertise, teaching experience, and professional development activities. A diverse and highly qualified faculty supports the program's mission and enhances student learning.

Faculty-to-Student Ratios

Faculty-to-student ratios are a key metric in this section. Research has shown that smaller ratios improve student outcomes, particularly in clinical settings. The *American Association of Colleges of Nursing* (AACN) recommends a ratio of 1:10 for clinical courses to ensure adequate supervision and guidance. Programs should provide evidence that they meet or exceed this standard.

Ongoing Professional Development

Faculty development is another critical aspect. Accrediting bodies expect programs to support faculty pursuing continuing education, certifications, and research opportunities. A well-documented professional development plan demonstrates the program's commitment to maintaining a competent and current faculty.

Curriculum Review and Alignment with Accreditation Standards

The curriculum is the heart of the nursing program and a focal point of the self-study. This section should detail how the curriculum aligns with accreditation standards and prepares students for professional practice.

Mapping the Curriculum

Programs should include a curriculum map that links courses to program outcomes and accreditation standards. For example, a pharmacology course might align with outcomes related to safe medication administration and evidence-based practice. Precise mapping ensures that students are adequately prepared for the NCLEX and future nurse roles.

Integrating Emerging Trends

Accrediting agencies also evaluate how programs adapt their curricula to reflect emerging trends in healthcare. For instance, the increasing emphasis on telehealth and population health management requires nursing programs to integrate these topics into their coursework. Programs should highlight any curriculum updates that address such trends.

Student Support Services and Outcomes

Student support services are critical to ensuring student success and retention. The self-study should detail the resources available to students, such as academic advising, tutoring, mental health counseling, and career services.

Retention and Graduation Rates

Accrediting bodies closely examine retention and graduation rates, as these are indicators of program effectiveness. According to the *National Center for Education*

Statistics (NCES), the average graduation rate for nursing programs in the U.S. is around 60%. Programs with rates below this benchmark should provide strategies for improvement, such as enhanced mentoring programs or early intervention for at-risk students.

Diversity and Inclusion Efforts

Diversity and inclusion are increasingly important aspects of accreditation. Programs should document efforts to recruit and support students from underrepresented backgrounds. This might include scholarships, mentorship programs, or partnerships with organizations that promote diversity in nursing.

3.3 Presenting a Coherent Narrative

While these components are vital, the self-study should present them as part of a unified narrative. Accrediting bodies value a cohesive document demonstrating how the program's various elements work together to achieve its mission and goals. For instance, the mission statement should flow logically into the program outcomes, which faculty qualifications, curriculum design, and student services should support.

The structure of the self-study document is critical to accreditation success. By addressing each component thoroughly and cohesively, nursing programs can present a compelling case for their quality and effectiveness. Programs that invest time and effort into crafting a well-structured self-study enhance their chances of accreditation and position themselves for sustained excellence in nursing education.

3.4 Collecting and Organizing Evidence: Data, Reports, and Assessments

The self-study process hinges on providing clear, verifiable evidence that a nursing program meets accreditation standards. Collecting and organizing this evidence is a critical step that requires meticulous planning, collaboration, and documentation. Accrediting bodies rely on this evidence to evaluate the program's effectiveness, outcomes, and adherence to best practices. This section explores the importance of evidence collection, methods for organizing data, and strategies for streamlining the process.

The Role of Evidence in Accreditation

Evidence serves as the foundation of the self-study document. Accrediting bodies do not base their evaluations solely on narrative descriptions; instead, they require objective data demonstrating compliance with established standards. This evidence might include program outcomes, faculty credentials, assessment results, and institutional policies.

For example, an accrediting agency may request:

- **Student Learning Outcomes (SLOs):** Evidence that students meet expected clinical skills, critical thinking, and professional ethics competencies.
- **Program Outcomes include** NCLEX pass rates, job placement rates, and alumni satisfaction surveys.
- **Institutional Support:** Data on financial resources, technology access, and administrative support for the program.

Types of Evidence Required

1. **Quantitative Data** Quantitative evidence includes measurable, numerical information such as:
   - **NCLEX-RN Pass Rates:** A key metric for nursing programs. According to the *National Council of State Boards of Nursing* (NCSBN), first-time test takers' national average pass rate was approximately 79.9% in 2021. Programs must demonstrate that they meet or exceed this benchmark.
   - **Graduation and Retention Rates:** Indicators of student success and program effectiveness. The *National Center for Education Statistics* (NCES) reports an average retention rate of 60% for nursing programs, serving as a benchmark for comparison.
   - **Faculty-to-Student Ratios:** Evidence that the program maintains recommended ratios, such as the *American Association of Colleges of Nursing's* (AACN) suggestion of a 1:10 ratio for clinical supervision.
2. **Qualitative Data** Qualitative evidence provides context and depth to quantitative data. Examples include:
   - Student and faculty testimonials describing the program's impact.
   - Case studies of community engagement or innovative teaching methods.
   - Faculty and student reflections on clinical and academic experiences.

3. **Documentary Evidence** Documentary evidence includes written records such as:
   o Course syllabi and curriculum maps.
   o Faculty résumés and certification records.
   o Policy manuals and strategic plans.

Steps in Evidence Collection

Step 1: Identify Requirements The first step is understanding the specific evidence required by the accrediting body. Each agency provides a detailed list of standards and associated evidence, which serves as a roadmap for collection.

Step 2: Assign Responsibilities Collecting evidence is a team effort. Assigning specific responsibilities to faculty, staff, and administrators ensures accountability and prevents duplication of effort. For example:

- Faculty might collect syllabi and course evaluations.
- Administrators may compile budget reports and institutional policies.
- Student services staff could provide data on tutoring utilization and support services.

Step 3: Centralize Data Collection Centralized data management is crucial. Using shared drives, cloud-based platforms, or accreditation management software can streamline the process. Tools like Taskstream or Weave provide templates and systems for organizing evidence in a user-friendly format.

Organizing Evidence Effectively

Accrediting bodies emphasize clarity and accessibility. Poorly organized evidence can lead to delays, misinterpretations, or even denial of accreditation. The following strategies can help:

1. Develop a Document Framework. Organize evidence into sections that mirror the accrediting body's standards. For example:

- Standard 1: Mission and Vision
- Standard 2: Faculty Qualifications
- Standard 3: Curriculum and Outcomes

Each section should include subfolders for specific types of evidence, such as data, reports, and policy documents.

2. Use Cross-Referencing Cross-referencing allows programs to avoid duplicating evidence. For example, faculty qualifications might appear under "Faculty Credentials" and "Program Resources." Clearly labeled references help reviewers navigate the document easily.

3. Annotate Evidence Adding annotations or summaries to evidence documents provides context and clarity. For instance, a curriculum map might briefly explain how each course aligns with program outcomes and accreditation standards.

Challenges in Evidence Collection

Programs often encounter challenges during evidence collection, such as:

1. **Data Gaps:** Missing or incomplete data can hinder the process. For example, suppose NCLEX pass rates are unavailable for certain years. In that case, the program must address the gap and provide alternative evidence of student success.
2. **Inconsistent Documentation** Variability in how evidence is documented across departments can lead to confusion. Standardizing templates and formats ensures consistency.
3. **Resistance to Data Sharing** Faculty or staff may hesitate to share certain information, such as course evaluations or budget reports, due to privacy concerns or misunderstandings about the accreditation process. Open communication and training can alleviate these concerns.

Strategies for Success

1. **Engage Stakeholders** Involve faculty, staff, and students in the evidence-collection process. Their insights and contributions can uncover valuable evidence that might otherwise be overlooked.
2. **Leverage Technology** Tools like Microsoft SharePoint, Google Drive, or specialized accreditation software to streamline evidence organization and sharing. These platforms allow real-time collaboration and version control.
3. **Conduct Periodic Reviews.** Regularly reviewing and updating evidence ensures accuracy and readiness for accreditation. Annual reviews of outcomes, policies, and curriculum alignment can prevent last-minute scrambling.

Case Study:
Success in Evidence Collection

A mid-sized nursing program preparing for CCNE accreditation faced challenges organizing its faculty credentials and curriculum data. The program implemented a centralized evidence management system, assigning specific roles to faculty and staff. They used Taskstream to create a digital repository, linking each piece of evidence to the appropriate standard. As a result, the program completed its self-study three months ahead of schedule and received full accreditation with commendation.

Conclusion

Collecting and organizing evidence is a pivotal step in the self-study process. By focusing on clarity, consistency, and collaboration, nursing programs can effectively demonstrate their strengths and address areas for improvement. Properly prepared evidence supports accreditation success and enhances the program's internal evaluation processes, ensuring continuous improvement in nursing education.

3.5 Engaging Faculty, Staff, and Students in the Self-Study Process

Accreditation is a collective endeavor that benefits from all stakeholders' diverse perspectives and expertise. Engaging faculty, staff, and students in the self-study process ensures that the final document is comprehensive and reflects the program's strengths and challenges. This collaborative approach strengthens the self-study and fosters a culture of accountability, transparency, and shared commitment to excellence in nursing education.

The Role of Stakeholder Engagement

Accrediting agencies often evaluate the inclusivity of the self-study process. They recognize that the input of faculty, staff, and students adds depth and authenticity to the evaluation. Each group brings unique insights:

- **Faculty** contribute their understanding of curriculum design, pedagogical strategies, and student performance trends.
- **Staff** provide data on institutional policies, student support services, and administrative processes.
- **Students** offer feedback on the program's impact on their learning experiences, professional preparation, and personal growth.

Why Engagement Matters

1. **Ensures Accuracy.** Involving multiple stakeholders reduces the risk of overlooking critical details. For instance, faculty can verify the accuracy of curriculum maps. At the same time, staff can confirm the availability and effectiveness of student support services.

Engagement Matters
➤ Accuracy
➤ Buy-in
➤ Transparency
➤ Narrative

2. **Enhances Buy-In** When stakeholders actively participate, they feel a greater sense of ownership over the process and its outcomes. This buy-in can be pivotal for implementing any recommendations or improvements that arise during accreditation.
3. **Promotes Transparency** Engaging all program levels demonstrates a commitment to openness and honesty, which accrediting bodies view favorably.
4. **Strengthens the Narrative** Firsthand accounts from faculty and students add qualitative depth to the self-study, enriching its narrative with real-world examples of the program's impact.

Strategies for Engaging Stakeholders

1. Form a Diverse Self-Study Committee. Creating a multidisciplinary team ensures that all perspectives are represented. The committee might include:

- Faculty from various specialties.
- Administrative staff members, such as academic advisors and data analysts.
- Student representatives from different cohorts.

A designated chair or coordinator can oversee the committee, facilitate meetings, and ensure alignment with the accreditation timeline.

2. Conduct Regular Workshops and Meetings. Workshops and meetings allow stakeholders to share ideas, discuss findings, and offer feedback. Effective sessions include:

- **Orientation Workshops:** Introduce the accreditation process and its significance.
- **Data Analysis Sessions:** Review program outcomes and identify trends.

- **Draft Review Meetings:** Allow stakeholders to critique and refine the self-study document.

3. Use Surveys and Focus Groups. Surveys and focus groups capture broader perspectives, particularly from students and staff who may not be directly involved in the committee. Questions might address:

- Perceptions of curriculum quality and relevance.
- Satisfaction with faculty support and teaching methods.
- Experiences with clinical placements and hands-on training.

Surveys should be anonymous to encourage honesty, and focus groups should be facilitated by a neutral party to ensure open dialogue.

4. Recognize and Address Concerns Stakeholders may be concerned about their roles, workload, or process. Addressing these proactively helps maintain engagement. For example:

- Faculty might worry about additional responsibilities. Clearly define expectations and offer workload adjustments if necessary.
- Staff may feel their contributions are undervalued. Acknowledge their expertise and emphasize their role's importance.

Examples of Stakeholder Contributions

1. **Faculty Contributions**
   - Reviewing course materials to ensure alignment with program outcomes and accreditation standards.
   - Providing evidence of professional development, such as conference attendance or certifications.
   - Documenting innovative teaching practices, such as simulation-based learning.
2. **Staff Contributions**
   - Supplying data on student retention, graduation rates, and job placement statistics.
   - Highlighting the impact of student support services, such as tutoring or career counseling.
   - Ensuring compliance with institutional policies related to diversity, equity, and inclusion.
3. **Student Contributions**
   - Offering testimonials about the quality of education and clinical experiences.

- o Participating in focus groups to discuss program strengths and areas for improvement.
- o Sharing feedback on faculty engagement and mentorship.

Challenges in Stakeholder Engagement

While stakeholder involvement is essential, it is not without challenges:

1. **Time Constraints:** Faculty, staff, and students often have competing priorities. Scheduling meetings or workshops that accommodate everyone can be difficult.
2. **Limited Awareness** Some stakeholders may lack familiarity with the accreditation process. Without proper orientation, they may struggle to contribute meaningfully.
3. **Resistance to Change** The self-study process often reveals areas for improvement, which can be met with resistance. Faculty may hesitate to revise courses, or staff might resist altering established workflows.
4. **Inconsistent Participation** Maintaining engagement throughout the lengthy self-study process can be challenging. Stakeholders may lose interest or motivation over time.

Overcoming Engagement Challenges

1. Provide Training. Training sessions will be held to help stakeholders understand the accreditation process and their role within it. These sessions can cover:

- The purpose and goals of accreditation.
- Specific accreditation standards and their implications.
- How stakeholder input influences the self-study document.

2. Offer Incentives. Recognize and reward participation. This might include professional development credits or recognition in faculty performance evaluations. For students, incentives could include certificates of participation or small stipends.

3. Communicate Regularly. Regular updates keep stakeholders informed and engaged. Use newsletters, emails, or a dedicated accreditation webpage to share progress and upcoming tasks.

4. Celebrate Milestones. Acknowledging achievements along the way boosts morale. Celebrate completing a draft section, gathering key evidence, or reaching a project milestone with team recognition or small events.

Case Study:
Collaborative Success

A nursing program at a small university faced challenges in engaging its stakeholders during the self-study process. To address this, the program implemented the following strategies:

- Hosted monthly lunch-and-learn sessions to discuss progress and solicit input.

- Created a shared digital workspace where faculty, staff, and students could collaborate.

- Organized a student-led focus group to gather feedback on clinical experiences.

These efforts resulted in a highly collaborative self-study process. Faculty appreciated the opportunity to showcase their teaching methods, staff felt their contributions were valued, and students provided insights that enriched the document's narrative. The accrediting body praised the program's inclusivity and awarded full accreditation.

Conclusion

Engaging faculty, staff, and students in self-study is essential for creating a thorough, authentic, and impactful document. By fostering collaboration, addressing concerns, and recognizing contributions, programs can harness the collective expertise of their stakeholders to achieve accreditation success. Moreover, this engagement lays the groundwork for a culture of continuous improvement, ensuring that the program remains responsive to the needs of its students and the nursing profession.

3.6 Common Challenges and How to Address Them

The self-study process is often one of the most demanding aspects of accreditation. It requires meticulous planning, data collection, and critical analysis. Despite its importance, programs frequently encounter obstacles that can hinder progress and compromise the quality of the final document. Understanding these challenges and implementing proactive solutions is essential for success.

Common Challenges in the Self-Study Process

1. **Data Gaps and Inconsistencies** A comprehensive self-study relies on robust and accurate data. However, many programs struggle with:
   - **Incomplete Data:** Missing information on graduation rates, faculty credentials, or student outcomes can create significant hurdles.
   - **Inconsistent Data Collection Methods:** Different departments may use varying methodologies, leading to conflicting reports.
   - **Outdated Records:** Programs may discover that key metrics are not regularly tracked or updated.

   Impact: These gaps can weaken the program's ability to demonstrate compliance with accreditation standards, leading to questions about the program's effectiveness and oversight.

2. **Limited Resources** Nursing programs often face resource constraints, including:
   - **Time:** Faculty and staff typically juggle teaching, research, and administrative duties, leaving little room for self-study tasks.
   - **Personnel:** Small programs may lack dedicated personnel to manage the self-study process.
   - **Financial Constraints:** Budget limitations may restrict the ability to hire consultants, purchase software, or provide training.

   Impact: Resource shortages can slow progress and compromise the quality of the self-study document.

3. **Resistance to Transparency** A self-study requires honest evaluation, which can be challenging for institutions hesitant to reveal weaknesses. This resistance can manifest as:
   - **Fear of Judgment:** Faculty and staff may worry about how accrediting bodies will perceive gaps or shortcomings.
   - **Defensiveness:** Programs may overemphasize their strengths while downplaying areas needing improvement.

   Impact: A lack of transparency can result in an incomplete or overly optimistic self-study, potentially jeopardizing accreditation.

4. **Engagement Challenges** While stakeholder involvement is critical, maintaining consistent participation can be complex due to:

o **Low Awareness:** Stakeholders may not understand the importance or role of self-study.
o **Competing Priorities:** Faculty, staff, and students often have other pressing responsibilities that limit their ability to contribute.

Impact: Limited engagement reduces the depth and diversity of perspectives in the self-study.

5. **Alignment with Accreditation Standards** Interpreting and aligning with complex accreditation standards can be daunting. Programs may struggle with:
o **Ambiguity:** Standards can sometimes be vague or open to interpretation.
o **Shifting Criteria:** Accrediting bodies occasionally update standards, requiring programs to adapt mid-process.

Impact: Misalignment can lead to critical omissions or misrepresentation in the self-study document.

Strategies to Overcome Challenges

1. **Addressing Data Gaps**
o **Audit Data Systems:** Conduct a thorough audit of existing data collection processes to identify gaps early.
o **Standardize Methods:** Implement uniform data collection and reporting procedures across departments.
o **Invest in Technology:** Use database management systems or accreditation software to streamline data tracking and retrieval.

Example: A nursing program implemented a centralized data management system that improved accuracy and reduced retrieval time by 30%, enabling a more efficient self-study process.

2. **Maximizing Resources**
o **Prioritize Tasks:** Develop a clear timeline and action plan to allocate resources effectively.
o **Seek External Support:** Apply for grants or partner with other institutions to share resources.
o **Leverage Internal Expertise:** Assign tasks to faculty and staff with relevant skills to maximize efficiency.

Example: A limited-staff program designated specific faculty members as "data champions," trained to manage data collection and analysis. This approach streamlined the process and reduced workload distribution issues.

3. **Fostering Transparency**
   o **Promote a Growth Mindset:** Emphasize that the self-study is an opportunity to improve, not a punitive exercise.
   o **Create a Safe Space:** Encourage honest dialogue about challenges without fear of blame or repercussions.
   o **Celebrate Strengths and Weaknesses Equally:** Highlighting both areas of excellence and improvement demonstrates integrity and a commitment to growth.

Example: A faculty workshop focused on "celebrating challenges" helped one program frame gaps as opportunities, resulting in a more balanced and honest self-study.

4. **Boosting Engagement**
   o **Provide Education:** Offer orientation sessions to explain the self-study process and its importance.
   o **Incentivize Participation:** Recognize contributions through awards, professional development credits, or stipends.
   o **Use Flexible Scheduling:** Accommodate busy schedules by offering virtual meetings or asynchronous contribution options.

Example: A program hosted "Self-Study Saturdays," where faculty and staff could work collaboratively over lunch, fostering camaraderie and increasing participation.

5. **Ensuring Alignment with Accreditation Standards**
   o **Review Standards Thoroughly:** Assign team members to specialize in specific standards, ensuring nothing is overlooked.
   o **Consult Experts:** Engage external consultants or attend accreditation workshops to clarify ambiguities.
   o **Conduct Mock Reviews:** Simulate site visits or peer reviews to test alignment with standards.

Example: A program hired an external consultant to conduct a pre-accreditation review, identifying minor misalignments that were corrected before the official submission.

Case Study:

Overcoming Common Challenges

A nursing program at a mid-sized university faced several challenges during its self-study process, including data gaps, limited resources, and low engagement. By adopting the following strategies, the program successfully addressed these issues:

Data Gaps: Partnered with the institutional research office to centralize and update records.

Resource Constraints: Applied for a state education grant to fund accreditation-related expenses.

Engagement: Organized focus groups with students and faculty to gather diverse input and increase buy-in.

The result was a comprehensive and accurate self-study document demonstrating compliance with all accreditation standards. The program received full accreditation and positive feedback for its collaborative and transparent approach.

Conclusion

Challenges are an inevitable part of the self-study process but are not insurmountable. Nursing programs can navigate these obstacles by proactively addressing data gaps, resource limitations, transparency issues, engagement challenges, and alignment with standards. When executed well, the self-study becomes a requirement for accreditation and a roadmap for continuous improvement and excellence in nursing education.

3.7 Conclusion

Chapter 3 explored the critical role of the self-study process in nursing program accreditation. It emphasized the importance of self-study as a reflective and evidentiary document demonstrating a program's alignment with accrediting standards. The chapter outlined how to structure the self-study, focusing on key components such as mission and vision statements, program outcomes, faculty qualifications, curriculum alignment, and student support services.

Collecting and organizing evidence was highlighted as a cornerstone of the self-study. This involves compiling data, reports, and assessments to substantiate claims. Engaging faculty, staff, and students is essential to foster collaboration and ensure diverse input.

The chapter also delved into common challenges encountered during the self-study, including data gaps, resource limitations, resistance to transparency, engagement difficulties, and alignment with accreditation standards. Practical strategies were provided to address these obstacles, from conducting data audits and centralizing information systems to fostering a culture of openness and encouraging broad participation.

Real-life examples and case studies demonstrated how effective preparation and strategic planning can turn challenges into opportunities for improvement. Ultimately, the chapter underscored that a well-executed self-study meets accreditation requirements and is a valuable tool for program enhancement and long-term success.

Key Terms for Chapter 3: Self-Study and Documentation

1. **Self-Study**

   A comprehensive, reflective process used to evaluate a nursing program's alignment with accreditation standards, including an analysis of strengths and areas for improvement.

2. **Accreditation Standards**

   Specific criteria set by accrediting bodies that nursing programs must meet to achieve and maintain accreditation.

3. **Mission Statement**

   A concise declaration of a program's purpose, values, and objectives, guiding its strategic goals and alignment with accreditation requirements.

4. **Vision Statement**

   A forward-looking statement that outlines a program's long-term aspirations and goals within the nursing education landscape.

5. **Program Outcomes**

   Specific, measurable goals related to student achievements, program effectiveness, and alignment with industry standards.

6. **Curriculum Alignment**

   The process of ensuring that a program's curriculum meets the educational and professional competencies required by accrediting bodies.

7. **Faculty Qualifications**

The credentials, experience, and expertise of faculty members must meet accrediting standards to ensure quality instruction.

8. **Student Support Services**

Resources and services provided to nursing students, including advising, career counseling, academic assistance, and mental health support, to foster student success.

9. **Evidence-Based Documentation**

Data and materials collected to support claims made in the self-study, including reports, surveys, assessments, and performance metrics.

10. **Stakeholder Engagement**

The active participation of faculty, staff, students, and other stakeholders in the self-study process to ensure diverse perspectives and comprehensive input.

11. **Data Management**

The systematic collection, organization, and analysis of information needed to meet accreditation standards and prepare the self-study.

12. **Gap Analysis**

A method of identifying discrepancies between current program performance and accreditation standards, guiding necessary improvements.

13. **Continuous Quality Improvement (CQI)**

An ongoing process of assessing and enhancing program elements to ensure long-term effectiveness and alignment with accreditation criteria.

14. **Peer Review Process**

A component of accreditation in which external reviewers evaluate the program's self-study and documentation to provide feedback and determine compliance.

15. **Assessment Tools**

Instruments and methods used to evaluate program outcomes, such as surveys, standardized tests, and performance metrics.

16. **Best Practices**

Established methods or techniques recognized for producing optimal results are used as benchmarks in self-study preparation.

17. **Transparency**

An organizational commitment to openness and honesty in reporting data and addressing challenges during the accreditation process.

18. **Resource Allocation**

The distribution of personnel, financial, and technological resources to support program objectives and meet accreditation standards.

19. **Accreditation Compliance**

The act of adhering to the specific requirements and standards established by an accrediting body.

20. **Documentation Audit**

A systematic review of records and evidence to ensure completeness, accuracy, and alignment with accreditation requirements.

End of Chapter 3 Questions

Multiple Choice Questions

1. What is the primary purpose of the self-study process in nursing program accreditation?
   - o A) To showcase the program's achievements to the public
   - o B) To evaluate the program's alignment with accreditation standards
   - o C) To create promotional materials for potential students
   - o D) To justify program funding to external stakeholders
2. Which of the following is NOT typically a key component of the self-study document?
   - o A) Faculty qualifications
   - o B) Program outcomes and goals
   - o C) Student engagement strategies
   - o D) Marketing budget
3. Which document outlines the nursing program's long-term goals and aspirations?
   - o A) Mission statement
   - o B) Vision statement
   - o C) Program outcomes
   - o D) Self-study report
4. When collecting evidence for accreditation, which of the following is MOST important?
   - o A) Collecting feedback from program graduates
   - o B) Ensuring that evidence is based on data and aligned with accreditation standards

- o C) Gathering promotional materials about the program
- o D) Submitting paperwork on time to the accrediting body
5. Engaging faculty, staff, and students in the self-study process is crucial because:
    - o A) It helps create a cohesive and inclusive process
    - o B) It makes the process more time-consuming
    - o C) It encourages competition between departments
    - o D) It reduces the amount of evidence needed for submission

True/False Questions

6. The mission statement is a short-term, tactical document focused on the daily operations of the nursing program.
    - o True
    - o False
7. A gap analysis is used to identify discrepancies between a program's current performance and the accreditation standards.
    - o True
    - o False
8. Faculty qualifications and resources are considered irrelevant to the self-study process as long as the program has adequate student enrollment.
    - o True
    - o False
9. Continuous Quality Improvement (CQI) is a strategy used to make improvements in a program even after it has received accreditation.
    - o True
    - o False
10. The self-study process is a one-time event and does not require updates after initial submission.
    - o True
    - o False

Short Answer Questions

11. Explain the role of program outcomes in the self-study process for accreditation.
12. What common challenges do nursing programs face during self-study, and how can they be addressed?
13. Why is it important to align a nursing program's curriculum with accreditation standards, and what methods can be used to ensure this alignment?
14. What types of evidence are typically collected to support a nursing program's self-study, and how is this evidence used in the accreditation process?
15. Describe the role of faculty, staff, and students in the self-study process and explain why their engagement is essential for success.

Fill-in-the-Blank Questions

16. The _____ statement defines the nursing program's purpose and guides its strategic planning.
17. The process of identifying discrepancies between a nursing program's current state and accreditation standards is known as a _____ analysis.

18. _____ is a key process that involves continuously assessing and improving program elements to ensure ongoing compliance with accreditation standards.

19. _____ documentation provides the evidence needed to support the claims made in the self-study report.

20. One of the challenges of the self-study process is ensuring that all collected evidence is _____ and consistent with accreditation standards.

Essay Question

21. Discuss the importance of the self-study process in achieving nursing program accreditation. In your answer, explain the key components of the self-study document, the role of data collection and evidence, and how faculty and staff engagement can contribute to the process.

Chapter 4
Site Visits and Preparing for Review

The accreditation process for nursing programs culminates in a site visit, an essential component where external reviewers assess the program's compliance with established standards. A successful site visit is a testament to the hard work, organization, and preparation the nursing program has invested in meeting and exceeding accreditation requirements. This chapter explores the role of the site visit in the accreditation process, how to effectively prepare for it, and the key aspects that ensure success during the review.

4.1 Understanding the Role of Site Visits in the Accreditation Process

The site visit plays a pivotal role in the accreditation process of nursing programs, serving as the moment when the self-study document prepared by the institution is put into practice. While the self-study provides a comprehensive written account of a program's strengths, challenges, and compliance with accreditation standards, the site visit allows accrediting bodies to verify these claims in person. The site visit, typically conducted by a team of experienced reviewers, offers a deeper, more nuanced assessment of the program's operations, faculty, students, and infrastructure, ultimately helping to validate the program's educational quality and effectiveness.

The Importance of Site Visits in Accreditation

Accreditation ensures that nursing programs maintain high educational standards, meet legal and ethical requirements, and prepare students for professional practice. The site visit is a critical part of this process as it allows reviewers to observe firsthand the extent to which a program meets those standards. For accrediting bodies, such as the *Commission on Collegiate Nursing Education* (CCNE) and the *Accreditation Commission for Education in Nursing* (ACEN), site visits are an essential tool for determining whether the program is delivering on its promises, such as ensuring student success, delivering a rigorous curriculum, and providing adequate resources and faculty support.

The accreditation visit goes beyond evaluating physical spaces and resources; it examines the program's broader culture, faculty and students' engagement, and the alignment of all components—curriculum, clinical experiences, student outcomes, and administrative support—towards the program's goals. It is an opportunity to see whether the nursing program fulfills its mission of providing high-quality nursing education.

Site Visit: A Verification and Validation Process

Site visits are not meant to be adversarial or punitive. Instead, they are a process of verification and validation. Reviewers come to the institution to understand how the nursing program is functioning in real life. They review the self-study and assess whether the information presented accurately reflects the reality of the program. Their task is to validate the data provided in the self-study and ensure that it aligns with accreditation standards and reflects the program's strengths and challenges.

This validation process ensures that nursing programs granted accreditation truly offer quality education that meets the needs of the healthcare sector. Accrediting agencies use the site visit to gauge whether the program produces competent graduates, is well-prepared for clinical practice, and meets the evolving needs of the nursing profession. For example, suppose a nursing program claims its students are prepared for practice in a specific area, such as critical care. In that case, the site visit team will want to see concrete evidence—such as curricula that support critical care education and clinical placements in relevant settings—that supports this claim.

Comprehensive Assessment During the Site Visit

During the site visit, the review team will assess a broad range of factors, including:

1. **Curriculum and Instruction**: The team will observe how effectively the curriculum is designed to meet the established standards of nursing education. They will evaluate whether the program offers a balance of theory and clinical practice that supports achieving its outcomes. They will also review course materials, syllabi, and assessment strategies to see if they are aligned with professional nursing standards and current healthcare practices.
2. **Faculty and Teaching Quality**: A key aspect of the site visit is evaluating faculty qualifications, teaching effectiveness, and professional development. Reviewers will meet with faculty to assess their credentials, experience, and ability to support students' learning and development. Faculty may also be observed in the classroom and clinical settings to assess their teaching techniques and student engagement. Faculty

development initiatives will also be examined to see if the program ensures that instructors have ongoing opportunities for growth.

3. **Clinical Learning Experiences**: The site visit team will examine the program's clinical partnerships, placements, and resources. A crucial part of nursing education is providing students with sufficient clinical hours in various healthcare settings, which allows students to gain hands-on experience and apply theoretical knowledge in real-world situations. The team will assess whether clinical sites are appropriately equipped, whether preceptors are adequately trained and whether students are exposed to diverse patient care environments.

4. **Student Support Services**: The accreditation team will evaluate how much the program supports student academic and personal success. This includes reviewing advising systems, tutoring services, mental health and wellness resources, and student engagement opportunities. The team will also review retention and graduation rates, ensuring that the program supports students in completing their education successfully.

5. **Resources and Infrastructure**: The site visit team will inspect the program's physical resources, including classrooms, simulation labs, libraries, and technology used for learning. These resources are essential for providing students with the educational tools they need to succeed in nursing school. Adequate resources reflect the program's commitment to creating a positive learning environment and ensuring students can access the tools and equipment necessary for their education.

6. **Program Outcomes and Evaluation**: The review team will assess how the program tracks and evaluates its effectiveness through key outcomes, including graduation rates, NCLEX-RN pass rates, and job placement rates. They will evaluate whether the program systematically collects student success data and uses it to make informed decisions about curriculum development, faculty recruitment, and resource allocation.

The review team comprehensively understands the program's overall quality through these assessments. The site visit is a hands-on process designed to corroborate the findings from the self-study and provide a holistic view of how the nursing program functions in practice.

The Site Visit Report: Key Findings and Recommendations

After the site visit, the review team will compile a report that details their findings. This report typically includes an evaluation of how well the program meets each accreditation standard, along with strengths, areas for improvement, and any recommendations for how the program can address gaps in compliance.

The site visit report is a key document for the program's accreditation decision. Suppose the program is found to meet the standards. In that case, the accrediting body may grant full accreditation, often for a specific period, such as 5 or 10 years, depending on the agency. However, if deficiencies are identified, the program may be granted provisional or conditional accreditation, with a specified timeline to address the issues raised.

The accrediting agency may sometimes recommend specific actions or improvements, such as revising the curriculum, increasing faculty development opportunities, or enhancing clinical placements. The nursing program must submit progress reports and evidence of corrective actions within a designated period, which will be reviewed during a follow-up visit or report.

The Role of Site Visits in Continuous Quality Improvement

Site visits also allow nursing programs to engage in continuous improvement. They provide an external perspective that can help programs identify blind spots, prioritize areas of improvement, and enhance the overall quality of education. Reviewer feedback is invaluable for programs striving for excellence and can serve as a roadmap for future improvements.

Furthermore, the accreditation process encourages nursing programs to be self-reflective and proactive. By regularly undergoing accreditation and site visits, programs commit to a cycle of self-assessment and quality assurance. This commitment to ongoing improvement helps ensure that nursing graduates are equipped with the knowledge, skills, and competencies to meet the challenges of a rapidly evolving healthcare landscape.

Conclusion: The Critical Role of Site Visits in Accreditation

Site visits are essential to the accreditation process, providing a comprehensive assessment of nursing programs and ensuring that they meet the rigorous standards set forth by accrediting bodies. These visits are a form of external validation and an opportunity for programs to engage in self-reflection and continuous improvement. With careful preparation and alignment with accreditation standards, a nursing program can turn its site visit into a valuable learning experience that benefits students, faculty, and the broader healthcare community. By understanding the purpose of site visits and their process, nursing programs can position themselves for success, ultimately achieving accreditation and maintaining a reputation for providing high-quality nursing education.

4.2 How Site Visit Teams Assess Compliance with Accreditation Standards

The role of site visit teams in the accreditation process is to critically evaluate a nursing program's adherence to the standards set by accrediting bodies. These standards ensure that programs effectively prepare students for competent, ethical, and evidence-based practice in the healthcare environment. During a site visit, teams systematically assess how well the program aligns with these accreditation standards, verifying claims made in the self-study and evaluating the actual operations of the program. The visit allows the team to interact directly with faculty, staff, students, and administrators to assess the true functioning of the program.

Understanding Accreditation Standards

Accrediting bodies such as the *Accreditation Commission for Education in Nursing* (ACEN) and the *Commission on Collegiate Nursing Education* (CCNE) establish rigorous standards that guide the assessment of nursing programs. These standards are divided into key categories: mission and goals, student learning outcomes, curriculum design, resources, faculty qualifications, clinical placements, student support services, and program evaluation methods. Site visit teams evaluate how well the nursing program meets or exceeds these standards.

For example, a nursing program's goals should align with the institution's overarching mission and the accrediting body's expectations. Reviewers will assess whether the program's objectives are clearly defined and achievable and if they adequately support the development of students into competent, professional nurses. In terms of curriculum, accrediting standards require that programs have a robust, up-to-date, and evidence-based curriculum that reflects current nursing practice and meets the needs of students in various learning environments.

Verifying Documentation and Data

Site visit teams begin their assessment by reviewing key documentation the nursing program provides. This includes the self-study report, program outcomes, faculty qualifications, curriculum maps, student performance data, and evidence of student support services. The self-study document is critical, providing a detailed overview of how the program meets accreditation standards. However, the site visit team will not rely on these documents but will seek evidence to verify the claims made.

The team will look for tangible evidence of standards being met in practice to assess compliance. For example, suppose the program claims to provide students access to high-quality clinical placements. In that case, the site visit team will review documentation such as affiliation agreements or memoranda of understanding (MOUs) with clinical sites, contracts with healthcare facilities, and clinical logs. They may also visit clinical sites to observe how students are prepared for practice and whether they work in various clinical settings that align with program goals.

Similarly, when evaluating faculty qualifications, the site visit team will verify that faculty members hold the appropriate degrees, certifications, and professional experience required by accreditation standards. The team will also assess whether faculty members are actively engaged in professional development to remain current with nursing practices. This may include reviewing evidence of faculty participation in continuing education, research, and conferences.

Direct Observations: Classroom, Clinical, and Student Interactions

While documents are crucial, site visit teams also directly observe key aspects of the program's operation. These observations provide valuable insight into how the program is functioning in practice. Reviewers will typically attend classes and clinical rotations to observe faculty interactions with students, teaching methods, and the quality of instruction provided. In classrooms, the team will evaluate the teaching strategies used by faculty, the engagement of students, and the integration of evidence-based practices into the curriculum.

In clinical settings, the site visit team will observe whether students are exposed to diverse patient populations and appropriate clinical situations. They will assess the role of preceptors in facilitating students' learning experiences and the clinical learning environment itself. Are clinical instructors providing sufficient feedback to students? Are students demonstrating the skills and competencies expected of them at their stage of education?

The site visit team will also observe the physical facilities, including classrooms, laboratories, simulation centers, and other learning spaces. The program's infrastructure is a critical component of accreditation, as nursing students require specialized equipment and learning environments to master the skills needed for practice. Observing the facilities allows the team to assess whether resources are adequate to support the program's curriculum and student learning.

Interviews with Faculty, Staff, and Students

Another key aspect of the site visit is engaging with stakeholders through interviews and focus groups. The site visit team will hold discussions with faculty, staff, and students to gather qualitative data on the program's operations and the experiences of those involved. These interviews provide a broader perspective on the program's effectiveness and offer insights into areas not readily apparent in documents or direct observations.

Faculty interviews are valuable for assessing how well faculty members understand and engage with the program's goals, curriculum, and outcomes. The team will inquire about faculty development initiatives, opportunities for collaboration, and how faculty assess and address student performance. They will also seek to understand faculty satisfaction and engagement, as motivated and supported faculty are key to the success of any program.

Student interviews are equally important, as they provide insight into the student experience and the program's impact on student learning and success. The site visit team will ask students about their academic experiences, access to resources, faculty support, and clinical experiences. They will also gather feedback on student outcomes, such as graduation rates, NCLEX-RN pass rates, and job placement rates, and how the program has prepared them for professional practice.

Staff members, including administrative personnel, student advisors, and clinical coordinators, will also be interviewed to assess the support infrastructure of the program. These staff members are key to the program's day-to-day operations and support students academically and emotionally. Their input helps the site visit team gauge the level of support available to students and identify any gaps or areas for improvement.

Assessing Compliance with Student Support Services

Accreditation standards require nursing programs to provide various student support services that facilitate student success. Site visit teams will evaluate the program's counseling services, tutoring resources, advising structures, career services, and other student support systems. They will review student retention, academic performance, and post-graduation employment data and assess whether support services align with student needs.

For instance, if the program struggles with high dropout rates or low retention, the site visit team will assess whether sufficient support structures are in place to address these challenges. This may involve examining the availability of academic advising, mental health support, and career counseling services and whether students actively utilize these resources.

Assessing Program Outcomes and Continuous Improvement

One of the most important aspects of compliance is the program's ability to demonstrate positive outcomes and a commitment to continuous improvement. Accreditation standards typically require programs to collect and analyze data on student performance, graduation rates, job placement rates, and NCLEX-RN pass rates. During the site visit, the team will assess whether the program has systems for tracking and evaluating these outcomes.

The team will also review the program's processes for using outcome data to inform program improvements. Are student performance results being analyzed and used to modify the curriculum? Are trends in job placement rates being used to adjust clinical placement sites or program offerings? Does the program engage in ongoing self-assessment to ensure it remains responsive to changing healthcare needs?

Conclusion: A Holistic Approach to Assessment

Site visit teams take a holistic approach to assessing compliance with accreditation standards, combining document reviews, direct observations, and interviews to form a complete picture of a program's effectiveness. By evaluating all aspects of the nursing program—curriculum, faculty, student outcomes, resources, and support services—the team ensures that the program meets the standards necessary to provide a high-quality education. This thorough process ensures that nursing programs continue to evolve and improve, ultimately producing graduates who are prepared to meet the challenges of the healthcare profession.

4.3 Preparing the Campus and Faculty for the Site Visit

Preparing the campus and faculty for a site visit is one of the most critical steps in the accreditation process. A successful site visit is not just the result of a well-documented self-study or favorable reviews of program data. Still, it is also heavily influenced by how well the campus and faculty are prepared to engage with the visiting accreditation team. This preparation requires careful planning, clear communication, and the active involvement of key stakeholders throughout the institution.

Communicating the Importance of the Site Visit to Faculty and Staff

One of the first steps in preparing for a site visit is ensuring that all faculty, staff, and stakeholders understand the significance of the accreditation process. It is essential to communicate that the site visit is not merely a formality but a rigorous evaluation that plays a crucial role in ensuring the program meets national and international standards for nursing education. Faculty and staff should understand that the accreditation process affects the nursing program's credibility, quality, and future.

To foster an understanding of the accreditation process, nursing leadership should host informational sessions or meetings to explain the purpose and goals of the site visit. This includes providing a clear overview of the accreditation standards, the self-study process, and what the visiting team will assess during their review. Faculty members should be encouraged to ask questions and provide feedback during these sessions, as their engagement and understanding will directly contribute to a smooth and successful site visit.

In addition to informational sessions, it is vital to outline the roles and expectations for faculty and staff members during the visit. This could involve assigning specific tasks, such as coordinating faculty interviews, organizing student focus groups, or preparing facilities for inspection. By making everyone feel involved and accountable, the preparation process becomes a collective effort that strengthens the institution's commitment to accreditation.

Preparing Faculty to Answer Questions and Engage with the Site Visit Team
One of the primary components of a site visit is interviews with faculty members. Faculty interviews provide the accreditation team insight into how the program is structured, aligns with accreditation standards, and how faculty members contribute to the overall educational experience. Nursing leadership should organize pre-visit training sessions or discussions to ensure faculty members are well-prepared for these interviews.

During these sessions, faculty should be briefed on what to expect during their interviews, including the questions the site visit team will likely ask. These questions may revolve around curriculum design, teaching methodologies, faculty qualifications, student assessment practices, and overall program goals. Faculty should be reminded that the purpose of the interview is not to critique individual performance but to assess the program's alignment with accreditation standards. Faculty members should be encouraged to be transparent and candid in their responses, providing specific examples of meeting the program's mission, goals, and objectives.

In addition to standard interview preparation, faculty should be aware of the importance of being prepared to discuss programmatic strengths and areas for improvement. Accreditation teams appreciate when faculty are reflective and aware of the program's limitations, as this shows a commitment to continuous improvement. Faculty members should be reminded to emphasize their contributions to the program's development, including course design, student engagement, and professional development efforts.

Faculty members should also be informed about the potential for site visit team members to observe their teaching through classroom visits or shadowing of clinical instruction. Ensuring faculty are prepared for this level of scrutiny allows them to present their best work, whether in the classroom or clinical settings. Faculty should be reminded to review their syllabi, lesson plans, and teaching materials before the visit to ensure alignment with accreditation standards and program outcomes.

Organizing Campus Resources and Facilities

Accreditation teams will typically visit the program's physical spaces, such as classrooms, laboratories, simulation centers, and clinical facilities. Preparing the campus involves ensuring these resources can be showcased during the site visit. This means ensuring that all spaces are clean, organized, and fully equipped with the necessary resources for learning.

Program administrators should coordinate with facilities management to ensure that the campus is in top condition on the day of the site visit. Classrooms and simulation labs should be equipped with relevant educational technology. Clinical facilities should be organized to demonstrate their role in the students' hands-on learning experiences. In addition to preparing the physical spaces, having the appropriate staff available to guide the site visit team through the facilities is crucial. It provides them with the context needed to understand how the resources are used in the program.

Nursing leadership should work closely with the program's simulation and clinical coordinators to ensure that these areas are prepared to demonstrate their role in student learning. For example, if a simulation lab is being reviewed, faculty members should be prepared to demonstrate how it is integrated into the curriculum and contributes to student competence in various nursing skills.

Faculty should also know that the team may want to observe the clinical placement process and visit some of the program's partner healthcare facilities.

Faculty and administrative staff should be well-versed in these relationships, including these partnerships' role in providing students with quality clinical experiences. Faculty should also ensure that their clinical instructors are prepared to discuss their contributions to student learning, including their assessment practices and feedback mechanisms.

Preparing Students for the Site Visit

While faculty are the primary participants in interviews and classroom observations, students also play an important role in the site visit process. Students will typically be asked to participate in focus groups or individual interviews with the site visit team, and they must understand the purpose of these discussions. Students should be informed about the importance of their feedback, as accreditation teams use student input to assess the program's effectiveness in preparing graduates for practice.

Nursing leadership should organize orientation sessions or meetings before the site visit to ensure students are adequately prepared. These sessions should cover the site visit, why the program seeks accreditation, and what students can expect during interviews or focus groups. Students should be encouraged to provide honest, constructive feedback on their experiences in the program, including aspects of the curriculum, faculty support, clinical experiences, and student services.

It is essential that students feel comfortable sharing their thoughts, as this provides accreditation teams with a real-world perspective on how well the program is meeting its goals. To facilitate this, students should be assured that their participation is voluntary and that their feedback will remain confidential. Faculty and administrators should encourage students to be open and provide specific examples of their experiences that will help the accreditation team understand the strengths and challenges of the program.

Logistics and Coordination of the Site Visit

Preparing the campus and faculty for a site visit also involves organizing the logistics of the visit itself. This includes coordinating schedules, arranging travel and accommodations for site visit team members, and organizing tours and interviews. It is essential to ensure that the site visit team has all the necessary information to conduct the review smoothly and efficiently.

A site visit schedule should be created in advance, with ample time for interviews, facility tours, and team discussions. This schedule should be shared with all faculty and staff involved in the visit, allowing them to prepare for their respective roles. For example, faculty who will be interviewed should be given advance notice so they can plan accordingly, and any logistical issues regarding transportation or access to campus facilities should be addressed ahead of time. Additionally, nursing leadership should designate a point person or coordinator who will serve as the primary contact for the site visit team and be responsible for managing any last-minute adjustments or concerns.

Final Preparations and Rehearsal

A week or two before the site visit, it is advisable to hold a final meeting or rehearsal to ensure everyone is ready. This is a time to review the schedule, assign any remaining tasks, and discuss concerns or questions. Faculty, staff, and students should feel confident in their roles and understand the expectations for their participation.

In this final review meeting, it is essential to review the key messages conveyed during the visit and ensure everyone is aligned on the program's strengths and areas for improvement. Faculty and staff should also be reminded to be professional, transparent, and collaborative during their interactions with the accreditation team. Nursing leadership can foster an environment of cooperation and success during the site visit by emphasizing the importance of presenting the program authentically and showcasing its strengths.

Conclusion

Thorough preparation for the site visit is a cornerstone of the accreditation process. Nursing programs can enhance their chances of a successful accreditation outcome by ensuring that faculty, staff, and students understand their roles and responsibilities and carefully coordinating the logistics of the visit. This preparation requires detailed planning, communication, and a shared commitment to the program's mission and goals. With a well-prepared campus, faculty, and student body, the site visit becomes a valuable opportunity to showcase the program's strengths and growth areas, ultimately leading to a successful accreditation review.

4.4 Coordinating Logistics: Scheduling, Tour Guides, and Communication with Visitors

Coordinating the logistics of a site visit is one of the most crucial tasks in the accreditation process, as the efficiency and professionalism of the visit reflect directly on the program's ability to manage resources and demonstrate its commitment to quality. A well-organized site visit ensures that the accreditation team can efficiently assess the program's compliance with standards while offering a smooth and positive experience for all parties involved. Proper logistical coordination involves scheduling interviews facility tours, providing clear communication, and ensuring that site visitors have all the necessary resources to complete their evaluation successfully.

Scheduling the Site Visit

The first step in coordinating logistics is establishing a clear and comprehensive schedule for the site visit. This schedule should be created as early as possible, ideally several months in advance, to ensure ample time for faculty, staff, and students to prepare. The schedule must detail each day's activities, including interviews, meetings, facility tours, and special sessions (such as student focus groups or public presentations).

A successful schedule balances the need for the accreditation team to gather detailed information with the time constraints of faculty and staff. When creating the schedule, program administrators should consider the availability of key faculty members, staff, and students who may need to participate in interviews or discussions. Ideally, a representative from each major program component should be available to discuss specific program elements, such as curriculum, student outcomes, assessment processes, faculty qualifications, and more.

The schedule should also provide ample time for the site visit team to tour key facilities, such as classrooms, laboratories, clinical sites, and other spaces supporting the program's educational mission. Time should be allocated to allow team members to observe teaching and learning in action, whether visiting a clinical placement site or sitting in on a simulation session or classroom lecture. Scheduling should also account for the necessary breaks and downtime for the site visit team, ensuring they do not feel rushed while navigating their assessments.

Once the schedule is drafted, it should be shared with all involved parties well before the visit to ensure everyone is prepared and can plan accordingly.

Flexibility is important, as site visit teams may require adjustments or have unforeseen needs that must be addressed quickly.

Designating Tour Guides and Campus Hosts

As the accreditation team will often need to tour campus facilities and observe the program's physical resources, it is essential to designate specific individuals as tour guides or campus hosts. These individuals will serve as the visiting team's primary contact points during their campus tour, ensuring that all the necessary information is communicated effectively.

Tour guides should be well-versed in the program's facilities and resources able to answer detailed questions about how the facilities support student learning and meet accreditation standards. For example, suppose a site visit team is touring a simulation lab. In that case, the tour guide should be able to explain how the lab is used in the curriculum, how faculty members are trained to use simulation, and how students are assessed in the lab. Similarly, tour guides should be prepared to discuss how clinical sites are selected, how student placements are managed, and how the facilities support patient safety and care quality.

In addition to guiding the site visit team through key locations on campus, hosts should provide context on the program's history, mission, and goals, helping accreditation team members connect physical spaces with the overarching goals of the nursing program. Program administrators should choose knowledgeable, well-organized, and approachable individuals, as the campus tour is an opportunity to demonstrate the professionalism and preparedness of the program.

The program should also designate backup hosts in case of scheduling conflicts or unforeseen circumstances, ensuring that the tour runs smoothly even if there are last-minute changes.

Effective Communication with Site Visitors

Effective communication with the accreditation team before, during, and after the site visit ensures a smooth process. Clear communication helps prevent misunderstandings, keeps the site visit on schedule, and ensures the visiting team has all the necessary information to conduct their evaluation.

Before the site visit, the program's leadership should establish open lines of communication with the accreditation team, introduce key contacts within the program, and share an outline of the visit schedule. A detailed itinerary should be provided in advance, including the names and titles of faculty or staff members involved in interviews or meetings. Suppose there are any changes to the schedule or facilities during the preparation period. In that case, it is critical to communicate these updates promptly.

Once the site visit begins, communication should remain clear and constant. Program administrators or a designated point person should be available to address any last-minute requests or concerns. This may involve ensuring that the site visit team has access to all needed rooms and facilities, addressing logistical concerns, or providing additional information.

The program must communicate openly about any potential challenges or limitations, such as faculty availability or specific aspects of the program that may not fully align with accreditation standards. Transparency will help foster an environment of collaboration with the accreditation team, allowing them to understand the challenges the program is facing and offering an opportunity for improvement.

One of the keys to successful communication is ensuring that all key stakeholders—faculty, staff, students, and administrators—are kept in the loop. Everyone involved in the site visit should be given clear instructions about where and when they are needed, their role, and how they can best contribute to the process. This clarity prevents confusion and enables the site visit team to gather all necessary information efficiently.

After the site visit, maintaining open communication with the accreditation team is equally important. Follow-up communications may be required if the team has additional questions or specific documentation needs to be provided. A post-visit debriefing meeting with key faculty and staff will allow the program to reflect on the visit, understand any areas for improvement, and prepare for future accreditation cycles.

Coordinating Student and Faculty Participation

One of the key aspects of the site visit is gathering feedback from students and faculty. Therefore, it is essential to coordinate their participation in the visit carefully. In addition to faculty interviews, the site visit team will often hold focus groups or individual interviews with students to gain insights into their experiences with the program.

Before the visit, nursing leadership should identify which students will participate in these sessions, ensuring that a representative cross-section of students is included. This means selecting students from various cohorts, levels of study, and clinical rotations to provide a comprehensive view of the program. Students should be briefed on the purpose of the focus groups and interviews, including the types of questions they may be asked and how their feedback will be used. Faculty members should also be informed about their roles in the site visit, with clear instructions on the types of questions they might be asked and any teaching or assessment materials they may need to present to the visiting team.

Faculty and student participation should be planned carefully to avoid scheduling conflicts. In addition, coordination with student services is necessary to ensure that students involved in the site visit are not disrupted in their academic schedules, allowing them to participate fully without interference in their ongoing coursework.

Conclusion

Coordinating logistics for a site visit requires attention to detail, clear communication, and proactive planning. Nursing programs can ensure the site visit process is efficient and effective by organizing a well-structured schedule, designating knowledgeable tour guides and campus hosts, and maintaining constant communication with all parties involved. Additionally, faculty and student involvement in the process should be carefully planned, ensuring their availability and preparedness to contribute to the accreditation team's assessment. By approaching the logistics of the site visit with professionalism and thoroughness, nursing programs can showcase their strengths, address any potential challenges, and ensure a smooth and successful accreditation process.

4.5 Preparing the Program's Key Stakeholders for Interviews and Discussions

Preparing key stakeholders for interviews and discussions during a site visit is pivotal to the accreditation process. These stakeholders—faculty, staff, administrators, and even students—are often the primary sources of information for the site visit team. As such, their ability to communicate effectively, present relevant data, and respond thoughtfully to questions plays a significant role in the outcome of the accreditation review.

Proper preparation of these individuals ensures that the program presents itself professionally and maximizes the opportunity to provide the accreditation team with accurate, thorough, and relevant information. With a thoughtful approach to preparing these stakeholders, nursing programs can demonstrate their commitment to continuous improvement, foster positive relationships with the accreditation team, and showcase how they meet or exceed accreditation standards.

1. Identifying the Right Stakeholders

The first step in preparing stakeholders for interviews is identifying who will be involved in the site visit discussions. Generally, the most important stakeholders to involve are those with direct knowledge of the program's core components, such as:

- **Program Leadership**: This includes the program director, department chairs, and other administrative leaders responsible for strategic planning, resource allocation, and overall program development. These individuals are essential for discussing the program's mission, goals, outcomes, and long-term plans.
- **Faculty**: Full-time and adjunct faculty members, particularly those responsible for core courses and clinical placements, play a central role in discussions around curriculum, instructional methods, assessment strategies, and student learning outcomes. Faculty must be prepared to explain their roles within the program, how they align with accreditation standards, and how they contribute to student success.
- **Staff**: Support staff members who manage student services, admissions, or faculty support systems should also be included in the preparation process. These individuals may be involved in discussions about student recruitment, retention strategies, advising, and the resources available to students throughout their educational journey.
- **Students**: Student participation is critical during the site visit, as they offer firsthand accounts of the learning environment, experiences with faculty, and access to resources. A representative sample of students should be selected to participate in focus groups or one-on-one interviews, ensuring that they are diverse in terms of year in the program, clinical placement, and background.

Each stakeholder group will need preparation tailored to their specific role in the program, ensuring that they can provide focused, meaningful responses to the accreditation team.

2. Understanding the Purpose of the Interviews

Before stakeholders can participate in interviews, explaining the purpose and expectations of the site visit discussions is essential. These interviews are opportunities for the accreditation team to assess compliance with standards and moments for stakeholders to reflect on the program's strengths and areas for growth.

Stakeholders must understand that the interviews aim to provide the accreditation team with a comprehensive, honest, and reflective program assessment. Stakeholders should be reminded that the interviews are meant to explore how the program meets accreditation standards and its ongoing efforts to improve quality. The program's leadership should emphasize that the accreditation team will be looking for evidence of the following:

- Alignment between the program's mission, vision, and curriculum
- Evidence of student learning and outcomes
- Faculty qualifications, performance, and development opportunities
- Resources and support systems available to students
- Continuous improvement strategies based on data-driven assessments

Reassuring stakeholders that the visit is not an evaluation of them personally but a broader review of the program will help alleviate anxiety and encourage honest, constructive conversations.

3. Preparing Stakeholders with Key Information

Each stakeholder group must be thoroughly prepared with the specific information they will be asked to discuss during the site visit. Program administrators should work with key stakeholders in advance to review relevant documents, data, and reports, ensuring they are familiar with the program's history, goals, and challenges.

For **faculty**, preparation involves understanding the program's curriculum in detail, knowing how course content and teaching strategies align with accreditation standards, and being able to explain how student outcomes are assessed. Faculty should be ready to describe the methods they use for teaching, how they incorporate best practices into the classroom, and how they respond to student feedback.

Program leaders and administrators should focus on the broader strategic objectives, such as how resources are allocated to support academic and student success, the program's long-term goals, and how data is collected to inform decision-making. Leaders should also be prepared to discuss partnerships with clinical agencies, community engagement efforts, and faculty development programs.

Students should be prepared to provide feedback on their experience in the program, focusing on factors such as the quality of instruction, availability of faculty, adequacy of resources, and the effectiveness of student support services. They should also be prepared to discuss their clinical experiences, opportunities for hands-on learning, and the program's support for professional development.

Topics the Review Team Will Focus On

Program Leaders & Administrators

- Strategic objectives
- Resources to support academic and student success
- How data is collected to inform decision-making
- Clinical partnerships
- Community engagement efforts
- Faculty development programs

Faculty

- Program's curriculum in detail
- Course content and teaching strategies align with standards
- How are student outcomes assessed
- How they respond to student feedback
- Professional development

Students

- Experiences in the program focusing on quality, faculty, resources, and effectiveness of student support services

Figure 6 Topics During Site Visits

4. Mock Interviews and Role-Playing

One of the most effective methods for preparing stakeholders for interviews is through mock interviews or role-playing exercises. These exercises allow stakeholders to practice answering potential questions, become comfortable with the process, and refine their responses before the site visit.

Mock interviews can be conducted by program leadership or with the help of external consultants familiar with accreditation processes. These practice sessions should include a range of questions that are likely to be asked during the site visit, including both factual questions (e.g., "How do you assess student learning outcomes?") and reflective questions (e.g., "What improvements have you made to the program based on student feedback?").

Mock interviews also help stakeholders learn how to manage difficult questions or situations. For example, suppose a stakeholder is unsure about the answer to a question or cannot recall specific data. In that case, they should be coached on how to respond diplomatically, such as offering to provide more detailed information after the interview or acknowledging challenges the program faces and sharing efforts to address them.

These exercises help stakeholders feel more confident and enable the program to fine-tune its overall messaging to ensure consistency and response alignment during the site visit.

5. Fostering a Collaborative Mindset

Preparing stakeholders involves providing specific information and cultivating a collaborative mindset among everyone involved. Site visits are a collective effort; everyone involved must understand the program's shared mission and the importance of presenting a unified front. Stakeholders should be encouraged to support one another throughout the process, ensuring that no one feels isolated or overburdened during the site visit.

For example, faculty should be prepared to discuss how their teaching practices contribute to the program's overall goals. Still, they should also be able to speak about how they collaborate with other faculty members to ensure curriculum coherence and consistency. Similarly, administrators should be ready to share how they support faculty development. Still, they should be prepared to demonstrate how they engage faculty in program decision-making and continuous improvement efforts.

This spirit of collaboration will create a more positive atmosphere during the site visit and show the accreditation team that the program is cohesive and committed to improving quality.

6. Providing Support During the Visit

Finally, preparing stakeholders also involves ensuring that they have adequate support during the site visit itself. This includes reminding them of the schedule and their roles, offering guidance if they feel uncertain during the interviews, and reassuring them to ask for clarification if any questions are unclear.

Establishing a support system for stakeholders during the site visit is important. For example, an internal contact person can be designated to assist with any last-minute questions or issues that arise, ensuring that stakeholders feel confident and prepared throughout the visit.

Conclusion

Preparing the program's key stakeholders for interviews and discussions during the accreditation site visit is a process that requires thoughtful planning and effective communication. By identifying the right individuals, providing clear instructions about the purpose of the interviews, offering detailed information, conducting mock interviews, fostering collaboration, and providing on-the-day support, nursing programs can ensure that their stakeholders are fully prepared to contribute to the accreditation process. The success of the site visit, and ultimately, the program's ability to achieve or maintain accreditation, depends significantly on how well these key individuals represent the program's strengths and address areas for improvement.

4.6 Common Pitfalls During Site Visits and How to Avoid Them

While site visits are critical in accreditation, they can also present challenges. These challenges may arise from misunderstandings, lack of preparation, or unforeseen issues that could negatively affect the outcome of the visit. However, by recognizing and addressing common pitfalls before the site visit, nursing programs can increase their chances of a successful review.

1. Inadequate Preparation of Stakeholders

One of the most significant challenges during a site visit occurs when stakeholders—faculty, staff, students, or administrators—are not adequately prepared for the interviews or the visit. Unpreparedness can result in incomplete or inconsistent responses, which can cause confusion for the site visit team and may raise concerns about the program's alignment with accreditation standards.

To avoid this pitfall, nursing programs must ensure that all stakeholders are prepared in advance. This involves conducting mock interviews, providing training on the standards the accrediting body will focus on, and ensuring stakeholders understand their roles and expectations during the visit. Faculty, for example, should be able to articulate how their teaching aligns with program outcomes, while students should be prepared to discuss their experiences in terms of curriculum, faculty interaction, and available resources. Administrators should also be clear on the program's strategic goals and allocation of resources.

Action Plan: Schedule regular review sessions with stakeholders to reinforce expectations and clarify any uncertainties. Encourage stakeholders to ask questions about their role in the process is unclear.

2. Misalignment Between Self-Study and Site Visit Observations

Another common pitfall is a mismatch between the information in the self-study document and what the site visit team observes during their time on campus. For instance, if the self-study claims certain resources or facilities are available to students, but the site visit team finds them inadequate or underutilized, it can raise doubts about the program's commitment to its goals.

This situation often occurs when programs are overly optimistic or fail to provide updated information in the self-study. For example, the self-study may highlight that students can access state-of-the-art simulation labs. Still, suppose those labs are outdated or lack the necessary equipment. In that case, it can create a disconnect between the program's claims and its actual practices.

To avoid this pitfall, programs must ensure that all claims in the self-study are accurate, supported by current data, and reflect the true state of the program. Administrators should internally review the self-study document before submitting it, verifying that all claims about resources, facilities, and student outcomes are up-to-date and substantiated by evidence.

Action Plan: Organize a review committee to double-check the alignment between the self-study and actual program practices, especially focusing on key areas like facilities, faculty credentials, and student outcomes.

3. Failure to Address Weaknesses and Areas for Improvement

Accreditation teams are tasked with evaluating not only a program's strengths but also its areas for improvement. A common pitfall is when programs fail to address known weaknesses or challenges during the site visit. For example, a program might have data that shows a low retention rate or issues with clinical placements. Still, suppose these issues are not addressed during the site visit. In that case, the accreditation team may perceive the program as unresponsive or unwilling to make necessary improvements.

Accrediting bodies value transparency and a commitment to continuous improvement. Programs that acknowledge their weaknesses and outline clear plans for addressing them are more likely to be viewed favorably. Failing to acknowledge or attempt to address weaknesses can lead to concerns that the program is not committed to improvement.

Action Plan: During the self-study and the site visit, be prepared to discuss areas for improvement openly and provide a clear action plan for how the program intends to address these issues. This can involve adjusting the curriculum, implementing additional faculty training, or improving student support services.

4. Inconsistent Documentation and Evidence

During the site visit, the accreditation team will expect to see substantial evidence supporting claims made in the self-study. If the program fails to provide the necessary documentation or if the documentation is disorganized, it can create doubts about the program's credibility and readiness for accreditation. For instance, the program may claim that it uses a particular assessment tool to evaluate student learning. Still, suppose the accreditation team cannot locate relevant samples or data to support this claim. In that case, it may result in concerns about the program's rigor or assessment processes.

Programs must be meticulous in gathering and organizing documentation to avoid this pitfall. All data, reports, assessments, and other relevant materials should be readily accessible and aligned with the accreditation standards. Organizing this evidence into specific categories that directly correspond to the standards being assessed is helpful.

Action Plan: Develop a well-organized system for collecting, storing, and labeling evidence. Create a central repository for accreditation-related documents and ensure all stakeholders can access and present them.

5. Lack of Engagement and Communication with the Accreditation Team

The accreditation team will conduct interviews and site tours, and their time on campus will be limited. A key pitfall is a lack of engagement or communication with the accreditation team, which can leave the site visit team feeling unsupported or unwelcome. This can also result in missed opportunities to clarify key issues or answer important questions that may arise.

To mitigate this risk, it is essential to maintain clear and open communication with the site visit team from the moment they arrive on campus. The program should designate a coordinator or liaison to facilitate communication between the visiting team and the program's stakeholders. This person should be available to assist with logistics, answer questions, and ensure the visit runs smoothly.

Action Plan: Assign a dedicated site visit liaison familiar with both the logistics of the visit and the program's content. This person should ensure that the visiting team has access to all necessary resources and support throughout the visit.

6. Over- or Under-Preparing for the Site Visit

Finding the right balance between over-preparing and under-preparing for the site visit is essential. Over-preparation can result in rehearsed, robotic responses from stakeholders, which may be inauthentic. Conversely, under-preparation can result in uncertainty and confusion, making it difficult for stakeholders to communicate the program's strengths and weaknesses effectively.

To avoid this pitfall, preparation should ensure stakeholders are well-versed in the key standards, comfortable with the process, and able to speak authentically about the program. This can be achieved by practicing mock interviews and reviewing key data points without over-coaching or scripting responses. Stakeholders should feel confident in their knowledge and have the flexibility to speak honestly, even about areas for improvement.

Action Plan: Focus on training stakeholders to be familiar with accreditation standards and the program's key performance areas, but avoid turning the preparation process into a rehearsed or scripted exercise. Encourage authenticity and transparency in all discussions.

7. Disorganization During the Site Visit

Finally, disorganization during the actual site visit can hinder the program's chances of success. This includes last-minute scheduling issues, missing materials, or confusion about where meetings occur. Disorganization can give the accreditation team the impression that the program lacks structure or is not fully committed to the process.

To prevent this, careful attention must be paid to logistics, such as scheduling meetings, preparing materials, and organizing tours. A clear schedule should be developed well in advance, and all stakeholders should be made aware of their roles and responsibilities during the visit. Designated individuals should ensure that materials are in place and that the accreditation team's needs are met promptly.

Action Plan: Develop a detailed site visit schedule and ensure all logistics are planned. Assign specific individuals to handle different tasks, such as managing meeting rooms, coordinating faculty interviews, and organizing tours.

Conclusion

By recognizing and addressing common pitfalls during site visits, nursing programs can ensure their accreditation process is as smooth and successful as possible. The key to avoiding these pitfalls is thorough preparation, clear communication, and a commitment to transparency and continuous improvement. When nursing programs can proactively manage potential challenges, they set themselves up for a positive review, demonstrating their readiness to meet accreditation standards and deliver high-quality education to their students.

4.7 Chapter 4 Summary

Chapter 4 focuses on the importance of site visits within the accreditation process and provides comprehensive guidance on how nursing programs can prepare for a successful site visit. The chapter explains site visits' critical role in accreditation, emphasizing how accreditation teams assess compliance with established standards.

The chapter delves into several key preparation strategies, including preparing the campus and faculty for the visit. Preparation involves ensuring all stakeholders— faculty, staff, students, and administrators—are informed about the accreditation standards and understand their roles. By conducting mock interviews and review sessions, programs can help ensure that stakeholders are well-prepared and that their responses align with the standards.

Logistical coordination is another central theme of the chapter. This includes scheduling the visit, organizing tours, and ensuring smooth communication with the accreditation team. Organizing the site visit effectively is essential to prevent delays or confusion, which could negatively affect the outcome.

The chapter also highlights the importance of preparing key stakeholders, such as faculty and administrators, for interviews and discussions during the site visit. Transparency and honesty during these interviews are crucial for presenting a program's strengths and areas for improvement.

Finally, the chapter addresses common pitfalls that programs may encounter during site visits. These include inadequate preparation, misalignment between self-study and site observations, failure to address weaknesses and disorganization. By recognizing these pitfalls and addressing them with thoughtful action plans, nursing programs can avoid common mistakes and improve their chances of success.

Chapter 4 provides a detailed roadmap for preparing nursing programs for site visits, emphasizing the importance of thorough preparation, clear communication, and organizational readiness to meet accreditation standards and demonstrate continuous improvement.

Key Terms for Chapter 4

1. **Site Visit**:
   A critical component of the accreditation process is where an external team of evaluators visits the program's campus to assess compliance with accreditation standards.

2. **Site Visit Team**:
   A group of experts and reviewers selected by the accrediting body to evaluate the program's compliance with accreditation standards during a site visit.

3. **Logistical Coordination**:
   The process of organizing all elements of the site visit, such as scheduling, arranging campus tours, and coordinating communication with the accreditation team.

4. **Stakeholders**:
   Individuals or groups with a vested interest in the nursing program include faculty, staff, students, administrators, and alumni.

5. **Mock Interviews**:
   Simulated interviews conducted in preparation for the site visit, designed to help faculty, staff, and administrators practice discussing the program's strengths, challenges, and outcomes.

6. **Self-Study Document**:
   A comprehensive document created by the nursing program before the site visit outlining the program's adherence to accreditation standards, strengths, and areas for improvement.

7. **Faculty Preparation**:
   The process of ensuring that faculty members are well-informed about the accreditation standards and are ready to engage in productive discussions during the site visit.

8. **Communication Plan**:
   A strategy for ensuring that all stakeholders involved in the site visit are kept informed about the process, timelines, and expectations, fostering transparency and smooth coordination.

9. **Site Visit Agenda**:
   A detailed schedule outlining the site visit activities, including meetings, interviews, and tours of the program's facilities.

10. **Accreditation Review**:

The overall evaluation process during which the accreditation team reviews evidence and documentation, including interviews and observations, to determine whether a program meets the required standards.

11. **Evidence Gathering**:

The process of collecting documents, reports, and data that demonstrate the program's compliance with accreditation standards. This may include student outcomes, faculty credentials, and curriculum reviews.

12. **Program Improvement Plan**:

A plan developed by the nursing program in response to feedback or areas for improvement identified during the site visit, demonstrating a commitment to continuous quality improvement.

13. **Transparency**:

Being open and honest about the program's performance, strengths, and challenges helps foster trust and credibility during the accreditation review process.

14. **Pitfalls**:

Common mistakes or challenges encountered during the site visit, such as poor preparation, miscommunication, or incomplete documentation, can negatively impact the program's accreditation outcome.

15. **Accreditation Outcomes**:

The results of the site visit, including whether the program achieves or maintains accreditation status and any conditions or recommendations for future improvement

End of Chapter 4 Questions

1. Multiple Choice Questions:

1. **What is the primary purpose of a site visit during the accreditation process?**
   - ○ a) To evaluate faculty performance
   - ○ b) To assess the program's compliance with accreditation standards
   - ○ c) To provide training for faculty and staff
   - ○ d) To collect tuition fees
2. **Which of the following is NOT a typical responsibility of the site visit team?**
   - ○ a) Evaluating the quality of the curriculum
   - ○ b) Interviewing faculty, staff, and students
   - ○ c) Providing funding to the program
   - ○ d) Reviewing the self-study document
3. **What is a key step in preparing faculty for a site visit?**
   - ○ a) Ensuring faculty are aware of accreditation standards and expectations
   - ○ b) Organizing a social event for the site visit team
   - ○ c) Encouraging faculty to avoid discussing the program with the accreditation team
   - ○ d) Asking faculty to write personal evaluations of their students
4. **Which of the following is an essential component of the logistical coordination for a site visit?**

- o a) Preparing the program's financial statements
- o b) Scheduling interviews and meetings with key stakeholders
- o c) Developing a new curriculum
- o d) Preparing marketing materials for the program

2. True or False:

1. The site visit team is responsible for creating the program's self-study document.
2. All stakeholders, including faculty, staff, and students, should be prepared to answer questions and engage in discussions during the site visit.
3. Preparing the program's facilities for a site visit is unnecessary, as the visit team will be familiar with the physical space.
4. Pitfalls during site visits, such as incomplete documentation or miscommunication, can negatively affect the outcome of the accreditation process.

3. Short Answer Questions:

1. Why is the site visit a critical component of the accreditation process?
2. How can a program prepare faculty for interviews during a site visit?
3. Describe one potential challenge during a site visit and how to avoid it.
4. What role does logistical coordination play in ensuring a smooth site visit?

4. Essay Questions:

1. Discuss the importance of transparency during the site visit and how it affects the program's evaluation.
2. Explain how preparing the campus, faculty, and key stakeholders for the site visit can contribute to a successful accreditation outcome.

Chapter 5
Meeting Accreditation Standards

Accreditation standards form the foundation for quality assurance in nursing education. They set the expectations for program performance, ensuring graduates are competent, prepared, and capable of addressing healthcare challenges. Adhering to these standards is not merely about compliance but embracing excellence and fostering a culture of continuous improvement. This chapter delves into the essential elements of accreditation standards, policy alignment strategies, data systems' role, and lessons from exemplary programs.

5.1 Exploring Key Accreditation Standards for Nursing Programs

Accreditation standards serve as a blueprint for nursing programs, outlining the benchmarks needed to achieve and maintain quality. These standards reflect the expectations of accrediting bodies and align nursing education with national and global healthcare needs. Key areas, including mission and goals, curriculum design, faculty qualifications, student support services, and program evaluation, form the foundation for program assessment and improvement.

Mission and Goals

A nursing program's mission articulates its purpose and reflects its commitment to addressing communities' healthcare needs. The mission must be clear, focused, and aligned with institutional priorities and broader public health objectives. Goals and objectives translate this mission into actionable and measurable outcomes, providing a framework for program success.

For example, a nursing program in a rural region might emphasize training nurses to serve underserved populations, with goals that include reducing the local nurse shortage by 15% within five years. This mission-driven approach demonstrates responsiveness to community needs. It aligns with standards set by accrediting bodies such as the *Accreditation Commission for Education in Nursing* (ACEN) and the *Commission on Collegiate Nursing Education* (CCNE).

A 2020 *American Association of Colleges of Nursing* (AACN) study highlighted the link between mission clarity and graduate outcomes. Programs with well-defined missions reported a 10% higher graduate employment rate within six months and a 15% increase in employer satisfaction ratings compared to programs with less cohesive mission statements. These statistics underscore anchoring program goals in a clear and relevant mission.

ACEN

- **Standard 1** Administrative Capacity and Resources
- **Standard 2** Faculty
- **Standard 3** Students
- **Standard 4** Curriculum
- **Standard 5** Outcomes

CCNE

- **Standard 1** Program Quality: Mission & Governance
- **Standard 2** Program Quality: Institutional Commitment & Resources
- **Standard 3** Program Quality: Curriculum and Teaching-Learning Practices
- **Standard 4** Program Effectiveness: Assessment & Achievement of Program Outcomes

Figure 7 Accrediting Agency Standards

Curriculum Design

The curriculum is the cornerstone of nursing education, blending theoretical knowledge, clinical competencies, and innovation. Accreditation standards ensure curricula are comprehensive, evidence-based, and aligned with national nursing competencies, such as the AACN Essentials.

THE ESSENTIALS:
CORE COMPETENCIES FOR
PROFESSIONAL NURSING EDUCATION

For instance, modern nursing curricula increasingly incorporate emerging fields like telehealth, population health, and interprofessional collaboration. Such updates prepare graduates to navigate a rapidly evolving healthcare landscape. Accrediting bodies require that these elements be woven into coursework and clinical training to ensure students are equipped for contemporary challenges.

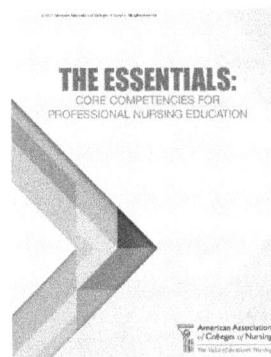

Figure 8 AACN Essentials.
https://www.aacnnursing.org/

Data from the *National Council of State Boards of Nursing* (NCSBN) illustrates the impact of curriculum alignment on outcomes. Nursing programs that integrated updated standards into their curricula reported a 92% NCLEX-RN pass rate, compared to an 87% pass rate in programs using outdated content. Furthermore, 85% of these programs observed enhanced critical thinking skills among graduates during clinical assessments.

Faculty Qualifications

Accrediting bodies emphasize the role of qualified faculty in delivering high-quality education. Faculty are expected to hold advanced degrees (master's or doctorate), maintain clinical expertise, and engage in professional development activities such as research, certifications, and continuing education.

Accredited programs often prioritize faculty development through institutional support. A 2022 AACN survey revealed that 78% of programs offered financial resources for faculty to attend conferences or pursue certifications. This investment fosters compliance with accreditation standards and enhances instructional quality. Faculty with advanced training often demonstrate higher teaching efficacy, as evidenced by improved student evaluations and increased student engagement in clinical settings.

Student Support Services

Support services are pivotal in student success, addressing academic and non-academic needs. Accreditation standards require programs to demonstrate how they provide resources such as academic advising, mental health counseling, and clinical placement assistance.

Effective support systems contribute to higher retention and graduation rates. Research published in the *Journal of Nursing Education* found that programs with robust student support services experienced a 15% higher retention rate and a 20% increase in first-time NCLEX-RN pass rates. These services are especially critical for nontraditional students, who often face additional challenges balancing education with personal responsibilities.

Clinical placement support is another critical area, as nursing programs must ensure students have access to diverse and high-quality clinical experiences. Accrediting bodies evaluate how well programs facilitate placements that align with curricular goals and prepare students for practice in various healthcare settings.

Program Evaluation and Continuous Improvement

Program evaluation is a dynamic, ongoing process that ensures nursing education meets evolving standards and student needs. Accrediting bodies require programs to collect and analyze data on key metrics such as:

- **Student Outcomes:** Graduation rates, licensure pass rates, and employment statistics.
- **Program Effectiveness:** Stakeholder satisfaction surveys and employer feedback.
- **Educational Quality:** Assessment of learning outcomes and faculty performance.

For example, a nursing program might analyze NCLEX-RN pass rates over five years to identify trends and implement targeted interventions. Continuous improvement processes, such as curriculum updates and resource allocation adjustments, help programs stay aligned with accreditation standards.

The importance of continuous evaluation is evident in a Midwestern nursing program case study, which increased its NCLEX-RN pass rate from 82% to 95% within three years by addressing gaps identified in its annual program evaluation. Key changes included revising pharmacology courses and introducing more clinical simulations.

5.2 Aligning Program Policies with Accreditation Requirements

Program policies serve as the framework that guides nursing education, operations, and compliance with accreditation standards. These policies cover all aspects of program management, including admissions, faculty qualifications, curriculum design, clinical placements, and student support services. Ensuring that these policies align with the rigorous expectations of accrediting bodies is essential for achieving and maintaining accreditation.

Understanding the Role of Policies in Accreditation Compliance

Policies are not merely procedural; they reflect the values and goals of the nursing program. For example, an admissions policy prioritizes diversity and equity, aligns with broader healthcare objectives, and meets the inclusivity requirements often emphasized by accrediting organizations like the *Accreditation Commission for*

Education in Nursing (ACEN) or the *Commission on Collegiate Nursing Education* (CCNE).

Accrediting bodies evaluate policies as part of the overall review process, assessing whether they support the program's mission and comply with accreditation standards. Noncompliance with a single policy area can jeopardize accreditation, making alignment a high-stakes endeavor.

Conducting a Policy Audit

The first step in aligning program policies with accreditation standards is a comprehensive policy audit. This process systematically reviews existing policies to identify discrepancies between current practices and accreditation requirements.

For instance, a policy audit may reveal that while the program requires 500 clinical hours, the accrediting body mandates a minimum of 600 hours. Similarly, policies on faculty qualifications may need to be updated to reflect requirements for advanced degrees or ongoing professional development.

Data from a 2021 study published in the *Journal of Nursing Regulation* found that nursing programs conducting annual policy audits were 25% more likely to achieve accreditation on the first attempt than programs with less frequent reviews. This highlights the importance of proactive and regular policy evaluations.

Collaborative Policy Development

Policy alignment is not a solitary task; it requires input from diverse stakeholders, including faculty, administrators, students, and external partners. Collaboration ensures that policies are both practical and compliant with accreditation standards.

Faculty involvement is particularly important. As individuals who implement policies in the classroom and clinical settings, their insights can help identify gaps and propose workable solutions. For example, faculty might recommend changes to clinical placement policies to reflect the realities of local healthcare facilities better.

On the other hand, administrators provide the institutional perspective, ensuring that policies align with broader organizational goals and resources. External stakeholders, such as clinical site representatives and alumni, can offer valuable feedback on how policies impact real-world practice.

Case Study:
Faculty Development Policy Revision

During a policy audit, a nursing program at a Midwestern university identified a gap in its faculty development policy. Accrediting standards required faculty to engage in professional development annually, but the program only offered sporadic opportunities.

The program revised its policy to include mandatory annual training sessions on emerging healthcare trends and pedagogical techniques. These sessions were supported through institutional funding and scheduled during breaks to maximize participation.

The results were significant: faculty survey scores on satisfaction with professional development opportunities increased by 20%, and student evaluations reflected improved instructional quality. The program also met accreditation requirements, praising its proactive approach during the site visit.

Aligning Admissions Policies with Accreditation Standards

Admissions policies are a critical area of focus. Accrediting bodies often require programs to demonstrate how their admissions processes support diversity, equity, and inclusion and the program's mission and goals.

For example, a nursing program that aims to address rural healthcare disparities might revise its admissions policies to prioritize applicants from rural backgrounds. This alignment satisfies accreditation requirements and advances the program's objectives.

Updating Clinical Placement Agreements

Clinical placements are integral to nursing education, and accrediting bodies scrutinize how these experiences are managed. Policies governing clinical placements must ensure that students gain exposure to diverse patient populations and settings while meeting the required number of hours.

Programs often collaborate with clinical partners to revise placement agreements. For instance, if a policy audit reveals that a clinical site no longer provides sufficient opportunities for pediatric care, the program may renegotiate the agreement or seek additional sites to fill the gap.

Continuous Monitoring and Improvement

Policy alignment is not a one-time task. It requires continuous monitoring to keep pace with changes in accreditation standards, healthcare trends, and institutional priorities. Many programs establish committees dedicated to policy review, ensuring timely updates.

For example, the COVID-19 pandemic prompted many nursing programs to revise their clinical placement policies to incorporate telehealth experiences. Programs with established systems for regular policy review could adapt quickly, ensuring compliance with accreditation standards while maintaining educational quality.

5.3 Developing Systems for Data Collection and Analysis

Data collection and analysis are essential components of accreditation preparation, serving as the basis for demonstrating compliance with standards, tracking program effectiveness, and identifying opportunities for improvement. Accreditation bodies increasingly emphasize data-driven decision-making, making robust systems for managing and interpreting data a critical requirement for nursing programs.

The Role of Data in Accreditation

Accrediting bodies require nursing programs to provide evidence-based documentation supporting quality and compliance claims. This includes data on student demographics, retention rates, NCLEX-RN pass rates, employment outcomes, and faculty qualifications.

For example, a nursing program might need to show that at least 80% of its graduates pass the NCLEX-RN on their first attempt, a common benchmark set by accrediting organizations like the *Accreditation Commission for Education in Nursing* (ACEN). Tracking such metrics becomes challenging without accurate and comprehensive data systems, potentially jeopardizing accreditation status.

In a 2020 survey by the *American Association of Colleges of Nursing* (AACN), 92% of respondents reported that robust data systems were critical to achieving accreditation, highlighting the necessity of this infrastructure.

Key Components of Effective Data Systems

1. **Data Collection**

Data collection begins with identifying the metrics accrediting bodies require and ensuring consistency across all collection processes. Common data points include:

- **Student Information**: Enrollment demographics, retention, and graduation rates.
- **Academic Performance**: Course grades, clinical evaluations, and licensure exam results.
- **Faculty Information**: Qualifications, professional development activities, and workload distribution.
- **Program Outcomes**: Employment rates, employer feedback, and alumni surveys.

Nursing programs often leverage existing platforms, such as student information systems (SIS) and learning management systems (LMS), to gather data efficiently.

2. Data Analysis

Collecting data is only the first step. Meaningful analysis transforms raw numbers into actionable insights. For instance, analyzing retention data can help identify at-risk student populations. Programs can then develop targeted interventions—such as tutoring, counseling, or mentorship programs—to address challenges.

A study published in the *Journal of Nursing Education* revealed that nursing programs implementing retention-focused initiatives saw retention rates increase by 30% among high-risk student populations. This underscores the potential impact of data-informed strategies.

3. Data Reporting and Visualization

Data reporting must be clear, comprehensive, and aligned with accreditation standards. Programs often use visualization tools like dashboards to present data in an accessible format for stakeholders. Charts, graphs, and summaries make it easier to identify trends, strengths, and areas for improvement.

For example, a program might create a dashboard displaying annual NCLEX-RN pass rates, retention statistics, and graduate employment outcomes. Such tools streamline internal reviews and impress accrediting teams during site visits.

Leveraging Advanced Data Systems

Modern technology has revolutionized how nursing programs collect, analyze, and report data. Integrated systems, such as LMS and SIS platforms, simplify the process by centralizing information in a single database.

According to a 2021 *National Center for Education Statistics* (NCES) report, 85% of accredited nursing programs in the United States use integrated data systems. These platforms offer several advantages:

- **Automation**: Automatically tracking metrics like student grades and attendance.
- **Real-Time Access**: Allowing faculty and administrators to access up-to-date data instantly.
- **Customization**: Tailoring reports to meet the specific requirements of accrediting bodies.

Cloud-based systems, such as Blackboard, Canvas, and PeopleSoft, are among the most popular tools used in nursing education. Their scalability and user-friendly interfaces make them particularly effective for managing large volumes of data.

Challenges in Data Collection and How to Overcome Them

Despite the benefits of advanced systems, nursing programs often face data collection and analysis challenges. Common issues include:

- **Data Silos**: Information stored in separate systems, making it difficult to access or integrate.
- **Resource Constraints**: Limited funding or staff expertise in managing complex data systems.
- **Human Error**: Inaccurate data entry or inconsistent reporting practices.

To address these challenges, programs can:

- **Adopt Interoperable Systems**: Ensuring platforms like LMS and SIS can communicate seamlessly.
- **Invest in Training**: Providing staff professional development in data management and analysis.
- **Conduct Regular Audits**: Verifying data accuracy and consistency through routine checks.

Case Study:
A Data-Driven Approach to Continuous Improvement

A nursing program at a large urban university faced accreditation challenges due to inconsistent data reporting. Student retention rates declined, and NCLEX-RN pass rates hovered at 76%, below the required 80% benchmark.

The program implemented a new data management system, integrating its LMS and SIS platforms. Faculty and administrators received training on data analytics, enabling them to monitor student performance more effectively.

Within two years, the program achieved the following results:

- **Retention Rates**: Increased by 12% due to targeted interventions for at-risk students.

- **NCLEX-RN Pass Rates**: Improved to 85%, exceeding the accreditation benchmark.

- **Graduate Employment**: Reached 90% within six months of graduation.

The program's use of data to inform decisions impressed accrediting teams, leading to full reaccreditation.

5.4 Lessons from Successful Programs

Learning from the strategies and successes of accredited nursing programs provides invaluable insights for other institutions aiming to meet accreditation standards. These real-world examples demonstrate the creative, resourceful, and mission-driven approaches that programs can adopt to align with accrediting body requirements while addressing unique challenges.

Urban Nursing Program: Advancing Diversity and Inclusion

Diversity and inclusion have become central themes in nursing education as the profession strives to meet the needs of increasingly diverse patient populations. One urban nursing program excelled by focusing on recruiting and supporting underrepresented groups, including racial minorities and first-generation college students.

Key Initiatives:

- **Targeted Recruitment:** The program partnered with high schools in underserved neighborhoods to promote nursing as a career option.

- **Mentorship Programs:** Incoming students were paired with faculty or senior students from similar backgrounds to foster a sense of belonging and academic support.
- **Cultural Competency Training:** Both faculty and students participated in workshops to build awareness and skills for addressing health disparities.

Outcomes:

- A 25% increase in graduation rates among minority students over five years.
- A commendation from the accrediting body for exceeding benchmarks related to diversity and inclusion.
- Higher levels of student satisfaction and alumni engagement, as measured by surveys.

This program illustrates how aligning institutional priorities with broader societal goals—such as addressing health inequities—can enhance compliance with accreditation standards while achieving tangible benefits for students and communities.

Rural Community College: Leveraging Local Partnerships

Rural nursing programs often face unique challenges, including limited financial resources and fewer opportunities for clinical placements. A rural community college overcame these barriers by partnering with local healthcare facilities, including small hospitals, clinics, and long-term care facilities.

Key Strategies:

- **Clinical Placement Agreements:** The program developed formal agreements with local healthcare providers, ensuring students had access to diverse clinical experiences.
- **Shared Resources:** Partnerships included using simulation labs and faculty exchange programs to supplement limited institutional resources.
- **Community Engagement:** The program involved community leaders and healthcare professionals in curriculum development to ensure alignment with local healthcare needs.

Outcomes:

- A 20% increase in clinical placement opportunities over three years.

- Graduate employment rates reached 95%, with most students securing jobs in their local communities.
- A significant reduction in program costs due to shared resources contributed to long-term sustainability.

This program demonstrates the power of community-focused strategies in addressing accreditation standards related to clinical training, resource management, and graduate outcomes.

Research-Focused Institution: Elevating Academic Excellence

Research-intensive nursing programs face challenges, including maintaining faculty engagement in research while ensuring high-quality instruction. One prominent institution successfully balanced these priorities by fostering a culture of evidence-based practice and academic scholarship.

Key Strategies:

- **Faculty Development:** The program provided competitive grants, conference funding, and sabbatical opportunities to encourage faculty research and publication.
- **Student Research Opportunities:** Undergraduate and graduate nursing students were integrated into faculty-led research projects, fostering a hands-on approach to evidence-based practice.
- **Interdisciplinary Collaboration:** Partnerships with other departments, such as public health and bioinformatics, expanded research opportunities and enhanced curriculum offerings.

Outcomes:

- Faculty publications increased by 40% over five years, strengthening the program's reputation.
- Accreditation benchmarks for faculty development were met and exceeded, earning praise from the accrediting body.
- Alumni surveys revealed that 85% of graduates felt well-prepared to incorporate evidence-based practices into their clinical work.

This case highlights how prioritizing faculty and student development can enhance compliance with accreditation standards while advancing the institution's academic mission.

Common Themes Across Successful Programs

Despite differences in focus, these programs share several key themes that contributed to their success:

1. **Alignment with Mission and Standards:** Each program ensured its initiatives aligned with institutional missions and accreditation requirements, creating a cohesive strategy.
2. **Stakeholder Engagement:** Faculty, students, administrators, and community partners were actively involved in the planning and implementation of improvements.
3. **Data-Driven Decision-Making:** Successes were guided by careful data analysis, allowing programs to identify areas for intervention and measure outcomes effectively.
4. **Innovation and Resourcefulness:** Programs leveraged partnerships, grants, and creative solutions to address challenges, demonstrating that even resource-limited institutions can achieve excellence.

Applying Lessons to Your Program

These examples provide a roadmap for other nursing programs seeking accreditation or reaccreditation. While each institution operates in a unique context, common strategies—such as fostering diversity, building partnerships, and supporting research—can be adapted to meet specific needs.

By learning from these success stories, nursing programs can enhance their ability to align with accreditation standards, improve student outcomes, and ultimately contribute to advancing the nursing profession.

Chapter 5 Summary

Chapter 5 outlined the essential strategies for nursing programs to meet and exceed accreditation standards. These standards provide a framework for maintaining high-quality education and producing skilled graduates to address evolving healthcare needs.

1. Key Accreditation Standards

Programs must address core areas such as mission and goals, curriculum design, faculty qualifications, student support services, and continuous program evaluation. Clear alignment with accrediting bodies' benchmarks ensures that programs remain relevant and effective. For example, integrating frameworks like the AACN Essentials strengthens curriculum design, while professional development for faculty enhances student outcomes.

2. Aligning Policies with Accreditation Requirements

Ensuring institutional policies comply with accreditation standards is crucial. Through audits and collaboration with stakeholders, programs can identify and address gaps. Adjustments, such as revising clinical hour requirements or faculty training protocols, help maintain compliance and improve program effectiveness.

3. Developing Data Collection Systems

Data collection and analysis are foundational to demonstrating compliance. Advanced systems, like learning management systems (LMS) and student information systems (SIS), streamline tracking metrics like retention and graduation rates. Effective use of data not only prepares programs for accreditation reviews but also enables targeted interventions that boost student success.

4. Lessons from Successful Programs

Real-world case studies highlighted diverse approaches to achieving accreditation. Urban programs emphasized diversity and inclusion, and rural programs leveraged local partnerships for clinical training, and research-focused institutions prioritized faculty development. These examples underscored the importance of innovation, stakeholder engagement, and data-driven strategies.

Conclusion

Chapter 5 emphasized that meeting accreditation standards is a dynamic process requiring a blend of compliance, creativity, and continuous improvement. By understanding key standards, aligning policies, utilizing data systems, and learning from successful practices, nursing programs can excel in accreditation and enhance their contribution to the healthcare sector.

Key Terms for Chapter 5

1. **Mission Statement**
   A formal declaration of a program's purpose, goals, and the values guiding its educational approach.

2. **Program Outcomes**

Specific, measurable achievements expected of students and graduates, such as NCLEX-RN pass rates or employment rates.

3. **Curriculum Design**

The structured content and sequencing of nursing program courses aligned with accreditation and educational standards.

4. **AACN Essential**

A framework provided by the American Association of Colleges of Nursing outlines core competencies for nursing education programs.

5. **Faculty Qualifications**

The academic and professional credentials required for nursing faculty to teach effectively and meet accreditation standards.

6. **Professional Development**

Continuous learning and skill enhancement activities for faculty to maintain expertise and improve instructional quality.

7. **Student Support Services**

Resources such as academic advising, counseling, and clinical placement assistance are designed to help students succeed.

8. **Program Evaluation**

The process of assessing a nursing program's effectiveness through metrics like graduation rates, retention rates, and job placements.

9. **Continuous Improvement**

Ongoing efforts to enhance a program's quality based on data analysis and stakeholder feedback.

10. **Data Collection Systems**

Tools and technologies, such as learning management systems (LMS) and student information systems (SIS), are used to gather and analyze data for program evaluation.

11. **Retention Rates**

The percentage of students who remain enrolled in a program over a specified period.

12. **Clinical Hours**

Practical, hands-on experience in a healthcare setting required as part of nursing education.

13. **Diversity and Inclusion**

Efforts to recruit and support individuals from underrepresented groups to create an equitable learning environment.

14. **Evidence-Based Practice**

The integration of research and clinical expertise to guide decision-making in nursing education and practice.

15. **Learning Management System (LMS)**
Software platforms used for organizing, delivering, and tracking educational content and student progress.

16. **Student Information System (SIS)**
A database system for managing student records, enrollment, performance, and outcomes.

17. **Case Study**
An in-depth analysis of a program or practice to highlight successful strategies and lessons learned.

18. **Compliance**
Adherence to the standards and regulations set forth by accrediting bodies.

End of Chapter 5 Questions

Multiple Choice Questions:

1. **Which of the following is NOT a key area covered by accreditation standards for nursing programs?**
    - o   A. Program mission and goals
    - o   B. Faculty qualifications
    - o   C. Faculty salary scales
    - o   D. Curriculum design and assessment
2. **What is the purpose of aligning a nursing program's mission with healthcare priorities?**
    - o   A. To ensure the program's financial sustainability
    - o   B. To guarantee high NCLEX-RN pass rates
    - o   C. To ensure the program remains relevant and responsive to community health needs
    - o   D. To attract more students
3. **Which of the following is an example of a program outcome?**
    - o   A. Faculty research productivity
    - o   B. NCLEX-RN pass rates
    - o   C. Number of clinical hours
    - o   D. Number of faculty certifications
4. **What is the primary reason for conducting a policy audit in the context of accreditation?**
    - o   A. To identify gaps and ensure alignment with accreditation requirements
    - o   B. To cut unnecessary expenses
    - o   C. To increase faculty workload
    - o   D. To determine student satisfaction levels
5. **Which data system is most commonly used to monitor nursing program outcomes and prepare for accreditation reviews?**

- ○ A. Excel spreadsheets
- ○ B. Learning Management Systems (LMS) and Student Information Systems (SIS)
- ○ C. Email surveys
- ○ D. Paper-based systems

True/False Questions:

6. **The program's mission statement should reflect the institution's goals and the evolving needs of the healthcare field.**
   - ○ True
   - ○ False
7. **Accreditation standards do not require nursing programs to provide evidence of student support services like academic advising or clinical placements.**
   - ○ True
   - ○ False
8. **Continuous improvement is a process that involves periodic reviews and adjustments based on data and stakeholder feedback.**
   - ○ True
   - ○ False
9. **Faculty members must only engage in professional development when first hired into the program.**
   - ○ True
   - ○ False
10. **The alignment of program policies with accreditation standards is essential for maintaining program quality and ensuring compliance.**
    - ○ True
    - ○ False

Short Answer Questions:

11. Why is curriculum design critical in meeting accreditation standards for nursing programs?
12. How do data collection systems, such as LMS and SIS, support accreditation efforts in nursing programs?
13. What are some common challenges programs face when aligning their policies with accreditation standards, and how can these be overcome?
14. Explain how a program's mission statement can contribute to its success in meeting accreditation standards.
15. Provide one example of a successful nursing program's strategy for improving student retention based on data analysis.

Discussion Questions:

16. Discuss how faculty qualifications and professional development impact the quality of nursing education and the program's ability to meet accreditation standards.
17. How can nursing programs ensure continuous improvement while maintaining compliance with accreditation standards?

18. How does the alignment of program policies with accreditation standards contribute to the overall effectiveness of the nursing program?
19. What role do student support services play in a nursing program's ability to meet accreditation standards? Discuss their importance.
20. Consider a nursing program in a rural or underserved area. What strategies could this program implement to meet accreditation standards while addressing the unique needs of its student population?

Chapter 6
Addressing Feedback and
Recommendations

6.1 How to Interpret and Respond to Accreditation Feedback

Accreditation feedback is an essential part of the evaluation process for nursing programs. It provides a snapshot of the program's strengths and areas where improvement is needed to meet national and regional standards. However, interpreting and responding to this feedback requires careful consideration and a strategic approach. Understanding the feedback process allows nursing programs to make informed decisions about how to move forward and to take concrete actions to align more closely with accreditation expectations.

Understanding the Structure of Accreditation Feedback

Typically, accreditation feedback is divided into three key categories: strengths, deficiencies, and recommendations. Understanding the purpose and context of each category is vital for crafting a meaningful response.

1. **Strengths:**
   Strengths highlight areas where the program excels and aligns with the accreditation standards. These positive aspects may include a well-established faculty development program, a strong curriculum design, or robust student support services. Accrediting bodies may also commend programs for being innovative in areas like interprofessional education or for their commitment to community engagement and diversity. Strengths often prove that the program is on the right track and reinforce practices that should be continued or further developed.

   Response:
   Programs should reinforce these strengths by maintaining the existing practices that were highlighted. It is also an opportunity to share these successes with internal and external stakeholders, demonstrating how the program meets or exceeds expectations. In some cases, programs may wish to expand upon their strengths to enhance the program's reputation and educational impact further.

2. **Deficiencies:**

   Deficiencies are the areas where the program does not meet the accreditation standards or has failed to address a specific criterion. These deficiencies often require immediate attention, as they could jeopardize the program's accreditation status. For instance, deficiencies may be identified in areas such as faculty qualifications, clinical placement hours, or assessment methods for student learning. Programs receiving deficiencies must act quickly to demonstrate that the program is taking corrective actions to address the issues raised.

   Response:

   The response to deficiencies must be timely and detailed. A program must create an action plan to address each deficiency, explaining the steps to resolve the issue. It is also important to designate who will be responsible for addressing each deficiency and set clear timelines for completion. Accrediting bodies often require regular updates on the program's progress in addressing deficiencies, so the program must track these changes carefully. Documentation of the steps to address deficiencies will be essential during re-evaluation.

3. **Recommendations:**

   Recommendations are areas where the program is not necessarily failing to meet accreditation standards but could improve to align better with best practices or emerging trends in nursing education. For example, accrediting bodies may recommend that programs integrate more advanced technology into the curriculum, offer more opportunities for clinical training in diverse settings, or provide additional faculty development resources.

   Response:

   Recommendations are generally non-binding, but addressing them can help improve the program's overall quality. These should be viewed as opportunities for growth rather than criticisms. The program should develop an action plan to address each recommendation, clearly identifying the steps for implementation. It is important to prioritize these recommendations based on the program's resources and long-term goals. When addressing recommendations, a program should focus on making sustainable improvements that will positively impact students and the community.

6.2 Assessing the Specificity of Feedback

Accreditation feedback can vary in terms of specificity. Some feedback may be very clear and specific, outlining exactly what needs to be changed. In contrast, other feedback may be more general and require further interpretation. Program leaders must dialogue with the accreditation body if the feedback is unclear. Clarifying any ambiguous points ensures that the program addresses the right issues.

For example, if the feedback indicates that the program's clinical placements need improvement but does not specify how the program should reach out to the accrediting body to ask for examples of best practices or additional guidance on what constitutes an appropriate clinical experience. This dialogue can help program leaders better understand the accrediting body's expectations and develop more targeted strategies for addressing the concerns.

Identifying Patterns and Priorities

When interpreting feedback, it is helpful to look for patterns. Suppose multiple deficiencies or recommendations, such as faculty qualifications or clinical placements, fall within a specific area. In that case, it may indicate that this area is a priority for improvement. By identifying trends or recurring themes in the feedback, the program can allocate resources effectively and ensure that its action plan addresses the most critical issues.

For example, suppose the feedback highlights deficiencies in clinical placements across several different accrediting reviews or mentions concerns about the availability of diverse clinical settings. In that case, the program may prioritize expanding clinical partnerships and exploring new healthcare settings to provide students with more diverse clinical experiences. This targeted approach can prevent the program from becoming overwhelmed by addressing every issue and ensuring that the most pressing areas are urgently addressed.

Developing a Systematic Response Process

Once feedback has been thoroughly interpreted, nursing programs must develop a systematic approach to respond to it. This process involves several steps:

1. **Forming a Response Team:**

    Forming a team of faculty, administrators, and possibly even students is essential to address the feedback. This team should analyze the feedback, develop action plans, and implement changes. Collaboration among various stakeholders ensures that different perspectives are considered, increasing the likelihood that proposed solutions are effective and realistic.

2. **Setting Priorities:**

Not all deficiencies or recommendations will require the same level of urgency. Some issues, such as updating course materials, may be relatively simple. In contrast, others may require more significant changes, such as overhauling the clinical experience structure. Establishing clear priorities helps program leaders focus resources and attention on the most critical issues first, minimizing the risk of delays.

3. **Creating an Action Plan:**

An action plan is a key part of responding to accreditation feedback. This plan should be detailed and specific, outlining the steps that will be taken to address deficiencies and recommendations. It should also include timelines, responsible individuals, and resources required to implement each action. The action plan should be continuously monitored and adjusted to remain on track.

4. **Documenting and Reporting Progress:**

Once the program has implemented the necessary changes, it is essential to document the process carefully. This documentation serves as proof of compliance and is crucial for re-evaluation. The program should prepare regular progress reports that outline the actions taken and the results achieved. These reports should be shared with the accrediting body and other stakeholders, such as faculty and students, to demonstrate that the program is committed to continuous improvement.

Responding to Positive Feedback

In addition to addressing deficiencies and recommendations, it is equally important to respond to positive feedback. Recognizing and celebrating the program's strengths boosts morale and fosters a culture of excellence. When the program is recognized for doing something well, it is an opportunity to highlight these strengths in promotional materials and accreditation reports, showcasing the program's high standards and its commitment to quality education.

Conclusion

Interpreting and responding to accreditation feedback is a dynamic process that requires critical thinking, collaboration, and strategic planning. Accreditation feedback is not just a report card but a valuable tool that enables nursing programs to enhance their quality and improve student outcomes. By interpreting feedback correctly, prioritizing actions, and developing a robust response plan, nursing programs can continuously evolve, strengthen their curriculum, improve faculty development, and better support their students, ultimately ensuring that they meet accreditation standards and remain competitive in the ever-evolving healthcare landscape.

6.3 Common Recommendations from Accreditation Agencies

Accreditation agencies provide valuable feedback on the areas where a nursing program may be deficient and through specific recommendations to improve the program's overall quality. While these recommendations are typically not mandatory, they represent best practices and emerging trends that can significantly enhance the program's effectiveness. Understanding common recommendations and proactively addressing them can improve student and program outcomes.

Recommendations for Program Mission and Goals

Accrediting bodies often recommend that programs revisit their mission and goals to align with current healthcare trends and workforce needs. This could involve adjusting the mission to reflect changes in healthcare delivery, such as a stronger emphasis on interprofessional education, community health, or global health initiatives. For example, a program might be encouraged to include a goal related to preparing nurses for leadership roles in managing health disparities in underserved populations, especially as the demand for healthcare professionals in rural or low-income urban areas grows.

In 2018, a study published by the *Journal of Nursing Education* highlighted the increasing trend of nursing programs aligning their missions with public health priorities. Programs that included goals focused on addressing health disparities saw a 12% improvement in NCLEX-RN pass rates and a higher graduate employment rate in public health settings.

Recommendations for Faculty Development

Accrediting bodies often recommend that programs improve their faculty development programs. These recommendations can range from increasing the frequency and scope of faculty training to enhancing opportunities for faculty to engage in research, clinical practice, or leadership development. Programs are frequently advised to ensure faculty maintains competency in teaching and clinical skills, particularly as nursing roles evolve with new technologies and treatment modalities.

One example is the recommendation for faculty to pursue certification in specialized areas of nursing. Accreditation bodies often encourage programs to ensure that their faculty are not only academically qualified but also well-versed in emerging fields, such as telemedicine or genomics, to keep pace with advancements in healthcare.

Recommendations for Curriculum Improvement and Innovation

Accreditation bodies frequently recommend curriculum review and innovation. These recommendations suggest that programs integrate contemporary healthcare issues into their curricula, such as mental health, substance abuse, telehealth, and cultural competence. As healthcare becomes increasingly complex, accreditation agencies emphasize the need for nursing programs to stay current with new treatments, technologies, and policy changes, ensuring students are equipped to provide the highest level of care.

A standard recommendation is for programs to incorporate more evidence-based practice (EBP) principles into their teaching. EBP is critical to improving patient outcomes, and accrediting agencies encourage programs to provide students with opportunities to critically evaluate and apply the best available evidence in clinical decision-making. Additionally, they may recommend including more interprofessional education (IPE) opportunities, where nursing students work alongside students from other healthcare disciplines, such as medicine, pharmacy, and social work, to simulate real-world team-based care.

In a 2020 *National League for Nursing* (NLN) survey, 57% of nursing programs implementing EBP-based curricula reported improved NCLEX-RN pass rates and graduate employment outcomes. Students trained focused on EBP were better equipped to navigate the complex clinical environments they would enter after graduation.

Recommendations for Clinical Placement and Experiences

Clinical placements are often a significant focus of accreditation feedback, with agencies recommending improvements in the quantity and quality of clinical experience offered to students. Accreditation bodies typically expect that students have access to various clinical settings to gain a broad range of experiences, including diverse populations, specialties, and healthcare settings.

Accrediting bodies often encourage programs to expand partnerships with healthcare facilities and community organizations to provide students with more robust, hands-on learning experiences. This may include clinical placements in underserved or rural areas, which can benefit the students' development and the local community. Agencies may also recommend that programs integrate clinical simulations into the curriculum to allow students to practice clinical decision-making in a controlled, low-risk environment before applying their knowledge in real-world situations.

For instance, a nursing program might be advised to increase students' hours in community health settings, including outreach to at-risk populations. This exposure enhances students' cultural competence and prepares them for the challenges they may encounter in diverse clinical environments. A 2022 report from the *Journal of Nursing Education and Practice* found that nursing programs that introduced more diverse clinical experiences had 15% higher retention rates and 20% higher employment rates for graduates than programs with limited clinical exposure.

Recommendations for Student Support Services

Accrediting agencies also provide recommendations to enhance student support services. These recommendations often involve improving academic advising, mental health support, career counseling, and mentoring programs. Accreditation bodies emphasize the importance of providing resources that support at-risk students, including those from underrepresented or non-traditional backgrounds, as these students often face more significant challenges in completing nursing programs.

One standard recommendation is the establishment of structured mentoring programs, where more experienced students or faculty provide guidance and support to newer students. Mentoring has been linked to increased retention rates, especially among minority and first-generation college students. According to the *National Advisory Council on Nurse Education and Practice (NACNEP)*, programs that implemented comprehensive student support structures reported a 17% improvement in graduation rates and a 12% improvement in NCLEX pass rates.

Additionally, programs may be encouraged to invest in technology supporting student learning and well-being. This includes virtual tutoring services, online peer support groups, and mental health apps. With the rising pressures of nursing education, addressing students' emotional and psychological well-being has become a critical component of accreditation recommendations.

Recommendations for Program Evaluation and Continuous Improvement

Lastly, accrediting bodies frequently recommend that nursing programs develop more rigorous processes for ongoing program evaluation and continuous improvement. This can include regular reviews of program outcomes, such as NCLEX-RN pass rates, graduation rates, and employment rates. Accreditation agencies encourage programs to use data from these reviews to identify trends, assess program strengths and weaknesses, and implement changes accordingly.

A common recommendation in this area is the establishment of formal, data-driven mechanisms for gathering feedback from alumni, employers, and current students. This feedback can help programs understand the effectiveness of their curriculum, teaching methods, and clinical placements. Based on this feedback, programs are expected to make improvements that reflect the evolving needs of the healthcare system and the workforce.

In 2020, a study by the *Council for the Accreditation of Nurse Anesthesia Educational Programs (COA)* found that programs regularly engaged in continuous program evaluation were 28% more likely to receive reaccreditation without conditions. Additionally, these programs showed improvements in student satisfaction and clinical competence.

Conclusion

Addressing recommendations from accreditation agencies is an important part of maintaining and improving the quality of a nursing program. While recommendations are generally not mandatory, they serve as valuable guidance for strengthening the program and ensuring it remains aligned with industry trends and educational best practices. By taking a proactive approach to address these recommendations, nursing programs can enhance their curricula, improve faculty development, increase clinical experiences, and provide better support for students, all while ensuring they are prepared for future accreditation reviews.

6.4 Developing an Action Plan for Addressing Deficiencies or Areas for Improvement

Once accreditation feedback is received, nursing programs must develop an action plan to address any identified deficiencies or areas for improvement. An action plan is critical for guiding the program through necessary changes and ensuring it remains compliant with accreditation standards. The plan serves as a structured roadmap that outlines how the program will make the required improvements and provides a timeline for implementing changes.

Understanding the Deficiencies

The first step in developing an action plan is to thoroughly understand the deficiencies or areas for improvement identified during the accreditation review process. Accreditation agencies often provide feedback in the form of detailed reports, including specific areas where the program has not met the expected standards. These deficiencies might relate to faculty qualifications, curriculum content, student outcomes, clinical placement hours, or support services. It is important for the program's leadership to carefully analyze the feedback and categorize the issues into specific themes, such as resources, processes, or student support.

For example, suppose the accreditation body notes that the program has not met faculty qualifications standards. In that case, the action plan will address faculty credentials through additional hiring, faculty development programs, or targeted certifications. Similarly, if student support services are deficient, such as inadequate clinical placement opportunities, the action plan will outline specific strategies to develop partnerships with healthcare facilities or enhance advising and counseling services.

Setting Clear and Achievable Goals

Once the deficiencies have been identified and understood, the next step is establishing clear, measurable goals for addressing them. Goals should be specific, achievable, and aligned with the accreditation standards. For example, if the accreditation feedback indicates that the program lacks diversity in its faculty, a specific goal might be to recruit at least two new faculty members from underrepresented groups within the next 18 months.

The action plan should include a timeline for achieving each goal. Establishing clear deadlines helps ensure accountability and provides measurable checkpoints for monitoring progress. The goals should also be prioritized based on their impact on program quality and the accreditation standards, with the most critical issues being addressed first.

For instance, if a nursing program's clinical placements are inadequate, the first goal might be to secure additional clinical rotation sites within the first six months of the action plan's implementation. Following that, the program could focus on expanding partnerships with community organizations to enrich clinical experiences further.

Identifying Resources and Stakeholders

An effective action plan will also outline the resources required to implement the necessary changes. This may involve securing additional funding, hiring new staff, or allocating time for faculty development. Resources could also include access to new clinical sites, technology for simulation labs, or curriculum development expertise.

Identifying key stakeholders is another essential step in the action-planning process. These stakeholders include faculty, administrators, clinical partners, students, and external consultants. Each stakeholder group will play a crucial role in implementing the plan. Faculty might be involved in curriculum revisions, while administrators could facilitate resource allocation or policy changes. Clinical partners may need to commit to offering additional clinical placements, and students may be required to provide feedback on proposed changes.

For example, suppose a program is aiming to expand its clinical experiences in underserved areas. In that case, the action plan may include reaching out to local community health clinics, forging partnerships with rural healthcare providers, and collaborating with faculty to design community-based learning experiences. Engaging stakeholders early in the process ensures that all parties are invested in the improvements and are aware of their responsibilities.

Designing Strategies for Implementation

Once goals and resources are identified, the next step is to design specific strategies for implementing the changes. This could involve creating new policies, revising existing curricula, or enhancing student support services. The implementation strategies should be realistic and aligned with the program's capacity. Sometimes, implementing all changes simultaneously may be overwhelming, so that a phased approach may be more effective.

For example, if a deficiency in faculty qualifications is identified, the action plan might outline the following phased strategy:

1. **Short-term (0-6 months):** Implement mandatory faculty development workshops focused on areas of need (e.g., advanced clinical practice, research methodologies).
2. **Mid-term (6-12 months):** Recruit additional faculty members who meet accreditation standards.
3. **Long-term (12-18 months):** Develop an ongoing professional development program for faculty that ensures continuous growth and adherence to accreditation standards.

Each strategy should include measurable milestones to assess progress. For instance, if the goal is to increase faculty diversity, milestones could include the number of candidates recruited, interviews conducted, and hires made within a set time frame.

Monitoring Progress and Adjusting

As the action plan is executed, monitoring progress and making continuous adjustments as needed is essential. Regular assessments of whether the planned changes are successfully implemented ensure the program stays on track. This could involve periodic meetings with key stakeholders to review the action plan's progress, track the completion of goals, and identify any barriers to implementation.

Data collection is an essential component of this process. For example, suppose the program improves student support services. In that case, it may track retention rates, student satisfaction surveys, or the number of students utilizing counseling or advising services. This data can provide insight into the effectiveness of the changes and indicate whether further modifications are necessary.

If a goal is not being met, the action plan should include strategies for troubleshooting and adjusting the approach. For example, suppose efforts to expand clinical placements fall short. In that case, the program might consider revising the strategy by seeking new clinical partners or offering virtual simulation experiences to bridge the gap.

Communicating Progress to Stakeholders

Effective communication is key to the success of an action plan. The program must regularly update all stakeholders on the plan's progress, the changes made, and the outcomes of those changes. Transparent communication builds trust and keeps everyone aligned with the goals.

For example, faculty should be informed about curriculum changes, and students should be notified about new academic resources or clinical opportunities. Administrators should be updated on the overall status of the action plan, including resource allocation. At the same time, external stakeholders, such as clinical partners or advisory boards, should be engaged in discussions regarding new collaborations or opportunities for program enhancement.

Documenting Improvements for Re-evaluation

As the action plan progresses, it is crucial to document all improvements and changes in preparation for future re-evaluation. Accreditation bodies will require evidence that deficiencies have been addressed and that the program meets accreditation standards. This documentation should include clear evidence of policy changes, improvements in faculty qualifications, curriculum revisions, and enhancements in student services. Documentation may include quantitative data such as NCLEX pass rates, graduation rates, employment outcomes, and qualitative data from student and faculty feedback.

By compiling thorough documentation, the program can demonstrate its commitment to continuous improvement and provide a comprehensive picture of the changes made. This will support the next accreditation review and enhance the program's ability to respond to future challenges and sustain its success.

Communicating Changes to Stakeholders (Faculty, Students, and Administrators)

Effective communication is crucial for successfully implementing an action plan that addresses feedback and recommendations from the accreditation review process. Clear and transparent communication ensures that all stakeholders—faculty, students, and administrators—are informed about the changes, understand their roles, and are motivated to support the process. In this section, we will explore how to communicate changes to each group, the importance of regular updates, and how to foster a culture of collaboration and continuous improvement.

1. Communicating with Faculty

Faculty members are integral to the success of any nursing program. They deliver the curriculum, mentor students, and contribute to program development. Therefore, engaging faculty early in communication is essential, especially when the program changes part of the accreditation action plan.

To communicate effectively with faculty, the program's leadership should hold regular meetings where updates on the progress of accreditation compliance are shared. These meetings should be an open forum where faculty can ask questions, express concerns, and provide input on the action plan's implementation. For example, suppose the accreditation feedback includes a recommendation to revise the curriculum to include more simulation-based learning. In that case, faculty should be informed of the proposed changes, their roles in implementing the curriculum, and the expected outcomes.

Providing clear, concise written communication in emails, newsletters, or memos is also important. Faculty members should receive documentation outlining specific changes, the timeline for their implementation, and the rationale behind the adjustments. For example, suppose changes to the faculty development policy are being made. Faculty should be informed about new continuing education or professional development requirements. This helps them understand how these changes align with accreditation standards and how they can contribute to the program's improvement.

Faculty development sessions or workshops may also be organized to support faculty in implementing the necessary changes. This could include training on new teaching methods, updated clinical standards, or changes in the program's assessment methods. When faculty see that changes are being implemented thoughtfully and that their professional growth is supported, they are more likely to engage with the changes and feel motivated to contribute to the program's success.

2. Communicating with Students

Students are the primary beneficiaries of a nursing program's accreditation process. They are often the group most directly affected by changes. Ensuring that students are well-informed about the changes and improvements is essential for maintaining trust and support throughout the accreditation process.

Communication with students should be transparent, timely, and clear. Regular updates should be provided through multiple channels, such as program meetings, emails, social media platforms, and the program's website. Suppose significant changes are being made to the curriculum, clinical placements, or student services (e.g., tutoring or counseling). In that case, students should be informed in advance to prepare for the changes.

For example, suppose the action plan includes revising the clinical placement process to offer more diverse healthcare settings or additional hands-on experience. Students should know how the new placements will benefit their learning and professional development. Additionally, if any changes in student policies or expectations arise—such as new attendance policies, additional clinical hours, or changes in assessment methods—students should be informed as soon as possible to avoid confusion or frustration.

In addition to formal communication, involving students in the process can help foster a sense of ownership and inclusion. Programs can establish student focus groups or surveys to gather input on the proposed changes and provide opportunities for students to ask questions and give feedback. This engagement helps students feel heard and provides valuable insights into how changes might impact their learning experience.

3. Communicating with Administrators

Administrators play a key role in supporting the accreditation process, as they are responsible for allocating resources, overseeing policies, and ensuring the program's overall success. For administrators, communication should focus on how the accreditation feedback aligns with institutional goals and how their leadership can support the program's compliance efforts.

Regular reports, meetings, and program leadership updates should inform administrators of progress. These communications should outline the action plan, provide status updates on implementing changes, and highlight any resource needs that may arise. For instance, if the action plan calls for updating technology or expanding clinical sites, administrators should be informed of the financial or logistical support required to achieve these goals. By understanding the broader goals and requirements, administrators are better equipped to advocate for necessary resources or policy changes.

Moreover, administrators should be engaged in the evaluation process, as their support is often critical to overcoming challenges and maintaining momentum. Suppose faculty or students encounter barriers to implementing the changes. In that case, administrators can provide guidance or reallocate resources to support the effort. A close partnership between program leadership and administrators will help to ensure the program stays on track toward meeting accreditation standards.

4. Fostering a Collaborative Environment

Effective communication is about conveying information and fostering a culture of collaboration and shared responsibility. Accreditation is a collective effort that requires the active involvement of all stakeholders. The more collaborative the process, the more likely the program is to succeed in meeting accreditation standards.

To foster this collaboration, program leaders should emphasize the importance of teamwork and encourage cross-functional communication. Faculty, students, and administrators should all understand that the improvements being made are for the benefit of the program as a whole and that their contributions matter. One way to facilitate this is by holding joint meetings or workshops where all stakeholders can discuss the changes, ask questions, and brainstorm solutions to potential challenges.

Program leaders should also be transparent about the accreditation process and its impact on the program's future. By sharing the long-term vision for the program's development, including how accreditation will improve the quality of education and student outcomes, stakeholders can feel more invested in the program's success. For example, sharing the positive outcomes from previous accreditation efforts—such as higher job placement rates or improved student satisfaction—can help motivate everyone to stay engaged and committed to the process.

5. Utilizing Technology for Communication

In today's digital age, utilizing technology is essential to communication. Tools like email, virtual meetings, and online platforms (e.g., learning management systems and student portals) allow for quick and efficient communication across multiple channels. Digital platforms can also enable real-time feedback, surveys, and virtual collaboration, making keeping all stakeholders updated and engaged throughout the accreditation process easier.

For instance, a nursing program might create a dedicated accreditation portal on the program's website where faculty and students can access updates, documents, and resources related to the action plan. Virtual town hall meetings or webinars could be held to explain the changes and answer questions, allowing for greater participation and interaction.

By leveraging technology, programs can ensure that communication is timely, efficient, and accessible to all stakeholders, regardless of location or schedule.

Conclusion

In conclusion, communicating changes to stakeholders is essential for ensuring the action plan's success and the nursing program's continued quality. When faculty, students, and administrators are kept informed, engaged, and supported, they can work together to implement the necessary changes and uphold the program's accreditation status. Clear, consistent, and transparent communication fosters a collaborative environment where everyone feels invested in the program's success and continuous improvement.

6.5 Documenting Improvements and Changes for Re-evaluation

One of the key components of a successful accreditation process is the documentation of improvements and changes made in response to accreditation feedback. This documentation records the program's efforts to address deficiencies. It is an essential tool for re-evaluation during subsequent accreditation reviews. Accurate, thorough, and well-organized documentation demonstrates the program's compliance with accrediting standards but also provides evidence of the program's ongoing commitment to continuous improvement.

The process of documenting improvements can be broken down into several critical steps, which we will explore in detail below.

1. Establishing Clear Documentation Practices

Before implementing any changes, it is essential to establish a clear system for documenting the process. This includes assigning responsibility for documentation, setting timelines, and ensuring that all stakeholders understand the importance of maintaining accurate records. Program leadership should designate a team or individual (such as the accreditation coordinator) to oversee this documentation effort and ensure it aligns with accreditation guidelines.

Documenting improvements requires more than just recording what has been changed—it involves tracking the rationale behind each change, the actions taken, and the outcomes expected. A comprehensive documentation system should include the following:

- **Timeline of Actions:** A clear record of when changes were implemented and when anticipated outcomes are expected. This timeline helps to demonstrate that the program has a structured and timely approach to meeting accreditation standards.

- **Detailed Descriptions of Changes:** A thorough explanation of the changes, why they were necessary, and how they address the recommendations or deficiencies identified in the accreditation feedback. For example, the accreditation review identified a need to improve faculty professional development. In that case, the program might document the introduction of new faculty workshops, the topics covered, and participant feedback.

- **Evidence of Implementation:** This includes records such as meeting minutes, training materials, curriculum syllabi, or student surveys. The more concrete the evidence, the stronger the case for re-evaluation. For instance, if a program introduced a new simulation-based learning component, the documentation should include curriculum changes, faculty training materials, and student feedback on the new teaching method.

2. Tracking the Impact of Changes

After implementing changes, tracking and measuring their impact is important to ensure they meet the desired outcomes. For example, suppose a program modified its clinical placement policies to improve student access to diverse healthcare settings. In that case, the program should document how the changes affected clinical training opportunities and student satisfaction. Tracking key metrics allows the program to gather the evidence to demonstrate effective and sustainable improvements.

Data collection methods could include:

- **Surveys and Focus Groups:** These tools can help gauge the perceptions of students, faculty, and clinical partners about the effectiveness of the changes. For example, a survey might ask students about their experiences with the new clinical placements or ask faculty about their perceptions of the faculty development workshops.

- **Assessment Data:** For programs that have made curriculum changes, collecting assessment data—such as exam scores, clinical evaluations, and student portfolios—can help demonstrate the impact of the changes on student learning outcomes.

- **Retention and Graduation Rates:** Changes to improve student support services, for example, can be tracked by looking at retention and graduation rates before and after the intervention. An increase in retention rates, especially for at-risk students, can strongly indicate that the changes are working.

- **Job Placement Rates:** Documenting employment outcomes can be a key success metric for programs with enhanced clinical placements or other career-oriented services. High job placement rates, particularly in underserved areas, can demonstrate that the changes improve graduate employability and address community health needs.

3. Ongoing Monitoring and Adjustment

Documentation of improvements should not be seen as a one-time task. Instead, it should be part of an ongoing monitoring and adjustment process. Programs must regularly review the impact of changes to ensure that they are achieving the intended outcomes and to identify any areas that may need further adjustment.

For example, if a program introduces a new student advising system but notices students still experiencing difficulties in academic planning, further revisions may be necessary. Documenting this continuous improvement process is essential for demonstrating to accrediting agencies that the program is committed to adapting to emerging needs and trends in nursing education.

Ongoing documentation helps create a feedback loop that ensures the program always works to enhance its effectiveness. This is a key part of the continuous improvement model, central to accreditation standards.

4. Preparing for Re-evaluation: How to Organize Documentation for Accreditation Reviews

When it comes time for re-evaluation during the next accreditation cycle, the program must be able to provide evidence that it has made improvements in response to accreditation recommendations. The documentation should be organized and accessible, ensuring the accreditation team can easily review it.

Programs can create a comprehensive portfolio or accreditation binder that includes:

- **A Summary of Changes:** This summary should highlight key improvements made since the last accreditation visit, including changes to curriculum, faculty development, student services, and assessment processes. It should also include the rationale for these changes and the intended impact.
- **Evidence of Compliance:** The portfolio should include evidence demonstrating how the program met the accreditation standards. This can include documentation of meetings, policies, student outcomes, and

other evidence showing the program's compliance with specific requirements.

- **Results of Assessments and Data:** The portfolio should include the results of assessments, student surveys, and performance data. This data proves that the changes have had the desired effect and improved program quality.
- **Stakeholder Involvement:** Accreditation bodies often seek evidence that faculty, students, and administrators were involved in implementing changes. The documentation should include records of meetings, feedback sessions, surveys, and any collaborative efforts made in response to accreditation recommendations.

By organizing the documentation, the program can present a compelling case demonstrating compliance with accreditation standards and a commitment to continuous improvement.

5. The Role of the Accreditation Coordinator

The accreditation coordinator plays a crucial role in documenting improvements and changes. This individual is responsible for gathering data, compiling reports, and submitting all required documents on time. To manage the documentation effectively, the coordinator must be organized, detail-oriented, and familiar with the accreditation process. They also serve as the point of contact between the program and the accreditation agency, ensuring that follow-up actions or clarifications are promptly addressed.

6. Finalizing Documentation for the Accreditation Visit

As the accreditation visit approaches, all documentation should be finalized and reviewed. This includes ensuring that all necessary evidence is in place, that any deficiencies identified in the previous visit have been fully addressed, and that the program's improvements are articulated. A final review should be conducted to ensure that the documentation presents a comprehensive picture of the program's ongoing commitment to quality and continuous improvement.

Conclusion

In conclusion, documenting improvements and changes is vital to the accreditation process. It serves as evidence of compliance and helps programs track their progress, adjust where necessary, and maintain a focus on continuous improvement. By taking a systematic, data-driven approach to documenting improvements, nursing programs can demonstrate their commitment to excellence and increase their chances of a successful accreditation outcome.

6.6 Strategies for Fostering Continuous Improvement in the Program

Continuous improvement is a cornerstone of the accreditation process. It ensures that nursing programs are not static but are constantly evolving to meet emerging educational, healthcare, and professional demands. Accreditation bodies expect nursing programs to engage in a cycle of self-reflection, data collection, and process refinement. Implementing continuous improvement strategies helps maintain accreditation and drives higher educational standards, better student outcomes, and enhanced community health services.

Fostering continuous improvement involves creating a culture of accountability, collaboration, and responsiveness. Below are key strategies that can help nursing programs cultivate a mindset of continuous improvement.

1. Cultivating a Culture of Feedback and Reflection

A key element of continuous improvement is the ability to self-reflect and receive constructive feedback from all stakeholders, including students, faculty, staff, alumni, and clinical partners. Programs should develop formal and informal mechanisms to gather feedback from these groups, ensuring that the voices of all stakeholders are considered in the decision-making process.

- **Student Feedback:** Regular student surveys and focus groups can provide valuable insights into teaching effectiveness, curriculum design, clinical experiences, and student support services. Programs should analyze this feedback and look for patterns or recurring issues that may need to be addressed. For example, a recurring theme in student surveys about insufficient clinical placements in specific healthcare settings could prompt the program to reassess its partnerships with clinical sites.
- **Faculty and Staff Feedback:** Faculty and staff play a pivotal role in the success of nursing programs. Regular faculty meetings, one-on-one check-ins, and anonymous surveys allow staff to share their thoughts on the program's strengths and weaknesses. Their input can help identify areas for improvement in curriculum delivery, faculty development, or operational processes.
- **Alumni and Employer Feedback:** Alumni are an excellent source of feedback about the long-term impact of a nursing program. They can provide insight into how well the program prepared them for the

workforce and offer suggestions for improvements. Additionally, employers can inform the program about skills gaps they've observed in new graduates, which can guide curriculum updates and faculty development initiatives.

Creating a culture that encourages open dialogue and feedback requires leadership to model responsiveness to critiques and to act on the information received. Program administrators must listen to feedback and demonstrate a genuine commitment to addressing it.

2. Data-Driven Decision Making

Effective continuous improvement is built on data. Nursing programs must use reliable, consistent data to track student performance, faculty qualifications, and program outcomes. The goal is not only to measure success but also to identify areas that need attention or adjustment.

- **Student Performance Metrics:** Programs should regularly review data on student success, including NCLEX-RN pass rates, clinical competency assessments, and graduation rates. If trends in this data indicate a drop in performance, such as a decrease in NCLEX pass rates, the program should analyze the data to identify the root causes and implement targeted interventions, such as changes to the curriculum or additional academic support.
- **Clinical Placement and Job Outcomes:** Employment rates and clinical placement feedback are important metrics for the program's impact. For example, tracking graduate employment outcomes can show whether the program's graduates are being successfully integrated into the healthcare workforce. If job placement rates are low, the program may need to strengthen partnerships with healthcare facilities or revise career services offerings.
- **Faculty Performance and Development:** Data on faculty performance—such as student evaluations, peer reviews, and teaching assessments—can highlight strengths and areas for improvement. Faculty development initiatives should be based on these assessments, ensuring faculty members have the resources and support to enhance their teaching skills and remain current with industry trends.

Collecting and analyzing this data allows programs to make informed decisions about changes to the curriculum, policies, and student support services. These decisions are more likely to lead to meaningful, sustained improvements than decisions made without evidence.

3. Engaging in Benchmarking and Best Practices

Benchmarking against other successful nursing programs is an effective strategy for identifying opportunities for improvement. Benchmarking involves comparing key program metrics, such as faculty-to-student ratios, clinical placement quality, or NCLEX pass rates, against those of peer institutions or national standards.

- **Peer Comparison:** Programs should regularly compare their performance to similar programs, particularly those highly rated or who have received accolades for innovation or excellence. This can be done by attending conferences, networking with peer institutions, and reviewing data published by accrediting agencies and national nursing organizations like the AACN. Benchmarking helps identify best practices, such as effective teaching methods or innovative student engagement strategies, which can be adapted to fit the program's unique context.
- **Use of National Standards and Guidelines:** Accrediting bodies provide national standards that nursing programs must meet but also offer guidance on areas of excellence and innovation. Programs should stay informed about national trends in nursing education, such as new competencies or technological advancements like simulation-based learning. By staying current, programs can proactively align their practices with industry changes and maintain relevance in an evolving field.

Benchmarking can also extend to clinical sites. For example, if a program is struggling with limited clinical placements, it could look to peer institutions that have successfully expanded their clinical networks and identify strategies that could be applied to its program.

4. Professional Development for Faculty and Staff

Ongoing professional development is essential for fostering continuous improvement in nursing programs. Faculty and staff must have access to opportunities for professional growth, whether through conferences, certifications, workshops, or advanced academic training. Investing in faculty development supports teaching excellence and strengthens the program's ability to meet accreditation standards.

- **Evidence-Based Teaching Practices:** Faculty development should emphasize evidence-based teaching methods and strategies that enhance student learning outcomes. This could include training on active learning, flipped classrooms, or using technology effectively in nursing education.

Research has shown that faculty who continuously learn are better equipped to teach and inspire their students.

- **Clinical Expertise and Research Engagement:** Nursing programs should prioritize faculty engagement with clinical practice and research. Faculty who remain active in clinical settings bring current, real-world experience to the classroom. At the same time, those involved in research contribute to advancing the profession and improving program quality. Encouraging faculty to publish research, attend professional conferences, and participate in clinical practice enhances the program's academic reputation and meets accreditation expectations.
- **Mentoring and Collaboration:** Faculty mentoring and peer collaboration can further support professional development. Programs should establish mentoring relationships where junior faculty are paired with experienced mentors to help navigate academic and clinical teaching. Collaborative teaching models, where multiple faculties work together on courses or clinical rotations, can enhance educational quality and provide faculty with broader professional experiences.

5. Leveraging Technology for Improvement

Technology can play a crucial role in fostering continuous improvement in nursing programs. From learning management systems (LMS) to data analytics tools, technology enables programs to track student progress, assess curriculum effectiveness, and support faculty development.

- **Learning Management Systems (LMS):** Many programs use LMS platforms such as Blackboard, Canvas, or Moodle to manage course materials, grades, and assessments. These systems allow faculty to monitor student progress in real-time, provide immediate feedback, and identify at-risk students early in the course. Additionally, LMS platforms allow consistent course delivery and enable faculty to collaborate more easily across different teaching sites.
- **Simulation Technology:** Advanced simulation labs are becoming increasingly common in nursing programs. These high-tech environments allow students to practice critical clinical skills in a safe, controlled setting. Using simulation, nursing programs can provide students with valuable hands-on experience and evaluate their clinical competencies without the risk to actual patients. As simulation technologies improve, nursing programs must integrate these tools into curricula to remain competitive and aligned with accreditation standards.
- **Data Analytics Tools:** Advanced data analytics tools enable nursing programs to track student performance, analyze trends, and make data-driven decisions about curriculum, teaching methods, and student

support. Programs can use these tools to identify patterns in retention rates, graduation rates, and NCLEX pass rates, among other metrics, and then adjust their approaches to improve these outcomes.

By leveraging technology, nursing programs can create more efficient, effective systems for tracking progress, assessing outcomes, and facilitating continuous improvement.

6. Implementing Systematic Reviews and Audits

Programs should regularly conduct systematic reviews and audits to evaluate their performance against accreditation standards. This could include reviewing curriculum effectiveness, clinical placement processes, student support services, and faculty qualifications. Such reviews should be scheduled regularly (e.g., annually or biannually) and involve key stakeholders in the program.

Systematic reviews help ensure that all aspects of the program are continually aligned with accreditation standards. Moreover, they allow the program to identify potential issues proactively before they become significant problems. The findings from these reviews should be documented and used to inform future program improvements.

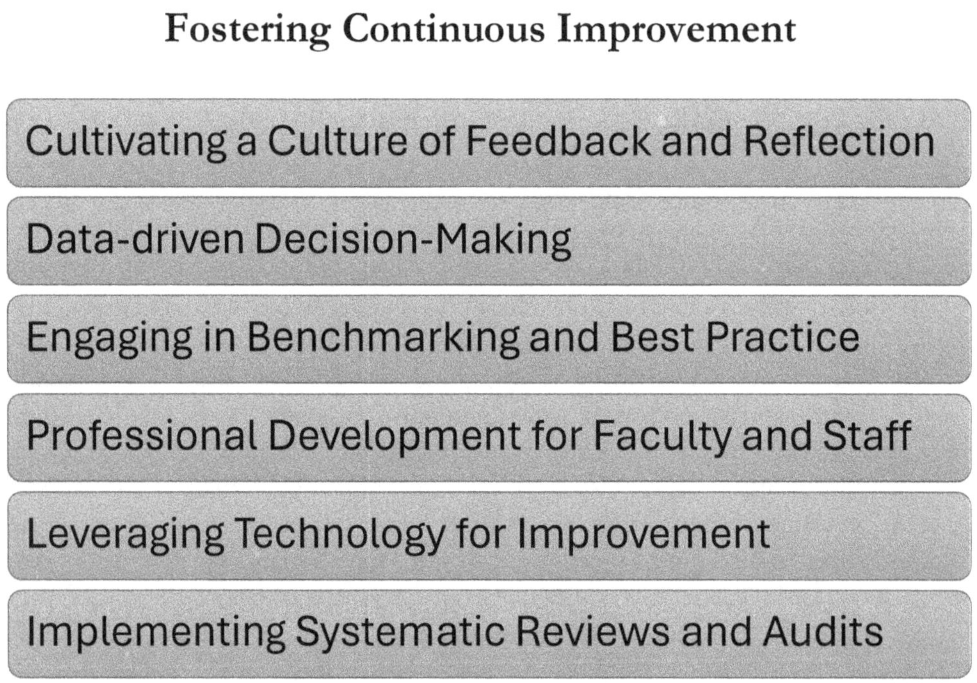

Fostering Continuous Improvement

Cultivating a Culture of Feedback and Reflection

Data-driven Decision-Making

Engaging in Benchmarking and Best Practice

Professional Development for Faculty and Staff

Leveraging Technology for Improvement

Implementing Systematic Reviews and Audits

Figure 9 Fostering Continuous Improvement

Conclusion

In summary, fostering continuous improvement in a nursing program requires a proactive, data-driven approach that involves engaging all stakeholders, using technology effectively, and prioritizing faculty development. By maintaining a culture of feedback and reflection, benchmarking against best practices, and tracking progress, nursing programs can ensure they meet accreditation standards and provide high-quality education that prepares graduates for success in the nursing profession.

Key Terms for Chapter 6

1. **Accreditation Feedback**:
   The evaluation and recommendations provided by accrediting agencies after reviewing a nursing program's performance in meeting established standards.

2. **Continuous Improvement**:
   A systematic approach to enhancing program quality through regular assessment, feedback, and iterative changes aimed at addressing deficiencies and enhancing student outcomes.

3. **Accreditation Deficiencies**:
   Areas in which a nursing program fails to meet the standards set by an accrediting body require attention and corrective action.

4. **Action Plan**:
   A structured plan to address identified deficiencies, including steps, timelines, and responsible parties for implementing improvements.

5. **Benchmarking**:
   The practice of comparing a program's metrics or practices to those of similar programs or national standards to identify areas for improvement.

6. **Data-Driven Decision Making**:
   The process of using collected data to inform decisions, track progress, and adjust program strategies and practices.

7. **Faculty Development**:
   Continuous learning opportunities and professional growth activities for faculty to improve their teaching practices and remain current in nursing education.

8. **Program Evaluation**:

The process of systematically assessing the effectiveness and quality of a nursing program, including curriculum, teaching methods, and student outcomes.

9. **Feedback Loops**:
The process of collecting, analyzing, and responding to feedback from various stakeholders helps programs improve their quality and performance.

10. **Self-Reflection**:
The practice of critically evaluating one's work and performance to identify strengths, weaknesses, and areas for improvement.

11. **Corrective Action**:

Steps taken to address areas of deficiency or non-compliance with accreditation standards are often guided by feedback from an accrediting agency.

12. **Quality Assurance**:
A proactive approach to ensuring that a nursing program maintains a high standard of education and continually meets accreditation criteria.

13. **Simulation-Based Learning**:
A teaching method that uses simulated clinical scenarios to enhance student learning and assess clinical competencies in a controlled environment.

14. **Stakeholder Engagement**:
Actively involving key stakeholders, such as faculty, students, and employers, in program improvement and decision-making.

15. **Program Review**:
A formal process in which a nursing program's effectiveness is evaluated based on data and outcomes to ensure continuous compliance with accreditation standards.

16. **Peer Review**:
The process by which faculty and administrators within or outside the institution assess a program's effectiveness and alignment with accreditation standards.

17. **Curriculum Mapping**:
The process of aligning the program's curriculum with accreditation standards and ensuring that it supports the achievement of student learning outcomes.

18. **Actionable Feedback**:
Constructive and specific feedback can be used to make tangible changes or improvements to the program.

End of Chapter Questions for Chapter 6

1. Why is interpreting accreditation feedback an essential part of the accreditation process, and how should a program approach the feedback received from accreditation agencies?

2. What common recommendations are provided by accrediting bodies to nursing programs, and why are these recommendations important for program improvement?

3. Explain the steps in developing an action plan to address deficiencies identified in accreditation feedback. What are the critical elements that should be included in this action plan?

4. How can nursing program administrators effectively communicate accreditation-related changes to faculty, students, and other stakeholders? What methods can ensure that all parties understand and implement the changes?

5. Why is documenting improvements and changes essential for re-evaluation during the next accreditation cycle, and what should this documentation include to be effective?

6. Discuss some strategies for fostering continuous improvement in a nursing program after receiving accreditation feedback. How do these strategies contribute to the program's long-term success?

7. What steps should be taken to develop a system for collecting and analyzing data related to accreditation feedback, and how can this data be used to make informed decisions about program improvements?

8. How can faculty and staff actively address feedback from the accrediting agency, and what best practices can encourage faculty engagement?

9. Why is it important to prioritize accreditation feedback based on its impact on program quality and compliance, and how can a program decide which deficiencies to address first?

10. How do continuous self-reflection and assessment play a role in addressing accreditation recommendations, and what practices can a nursing program adopt to foster a culture of self-improvement and responsiveness to feedback?

Chapter 7
Maintaining Accreditation Post-Approval

Once a nursing program achieves accreditation, the next challenge is maintaining that status. Accreditation is not a one-time event but an ongoing process that requires constant attention, adaptation, and improvement. The maintenance of accreditation ensures that a program consistently meets high standards of quality, directly influencing its reputation, student outcomes, and ability to provide exceptional nursing education. This chapter delves into the various components necessary to maintain accreditation, including understanding accreditation timelines, preparing for periodic reports, developing systems for quality assurance, engaging stakeholders, and staying updated with accreditation standards.

7.1 Understanding the Ongoing Accreditation Process and Timelines

While accreditation is a significant accomplishment for any nursing program, it is only the beginning of a continuous process that requires vigilance and ongoing compliance. Accreditation is not static, and programs must prove their continued adherence to national and regional standards through periodic reporting and reevaluation.

Typically, submitting a progress report is the first major milestone after initial accreditation. This report provides the accrediting agency with updates on the program's progress, addresses any deficiencies identified during the previous review, and ensures that the program remains aligned with accreditation standards. These progress reports are typically due one or two years after the program receives initial accreditation.

For instance, programs accredited by the *Accreditation Commission for Education in Nursing* (ACEN) or the *Commission on Collegiate Nursing Education* (CCNE) must submit comprehensive self-study reports every 5 to 10 years, depending on the accrediting agency's specific requirements. These self-study reports must present data on student outcomes, faculty qualifications, curriculum quality, and any changes in response to feedback from previous evaluations. Preparing such reports requires meticulous attention to detail and comprehensive data collection to demonstrate that the program is continuously meeting or exceeding accreditation standards.

The timing of accreditation reviews is crucial. Programs must remain proactive and continuously track compliance to avoid last-minute scrambles when submitting reports. This ongoing process requires institutional knowledge and careful planning, ensuring the program remains in good standing throughout the accreditation cycle.

Preparing for Periodic Reports and Reaccreditation Cycles

One of the most critical aspects of maintaining accreditation is preparing for periodic reports and reaccreditation cycles. Programs must collect data on key performance indicators during each accreditation cycle, including student retention rates, NCLEX-RN pass rates, graduation rates, and employment outcomes, to provide evidence of program effectiveness. This data should reflect success and highlight areas where the program continuously improves.

Reaccreditation cycles offer a valuable opportunity to demonstrate the program's growth and address any deficiencies that may have been identified in prior evaluations. Suppose a program's previous report noted insufficient clinical placements or faculty development was lacking. In that case, the program must present evidence of how these issues have been addressed during the reaccreditation process.

Program administrators should collaborate with faculty and staff to review data and performance metrics to prepare for these cycles, ensuring any discrepancies are addressed. Feedback from stakeholders—such as students, alumni, clinical partners, and employers—can also provide valuable insights into areas where the program may need to improve. In the case of nursing programs, feedback from healthcare employers can shed light on the skills and competencies needed in the workforce and help ensure that the program is adapting its curriculum to meet the evolving needs of the healthcare system.

Preparing for reaccreditation also includes a comprehensive review of the program's mission and goals to ensure they align with the current healthcare landscape. This might involve revisiting program objectives to ensure they address emerging trends in nursing practice, such as telemedicine, interprofessional collaboration, or integrating new technologies in patient care.

Establishing an Internal Review Process for Ongoing Quality Assurance

One of the most important aspects of maintaining accreditation is establishing an internal review process for ongoing quality assurance. This ensures that the nursing program complies with accreditation standards throughout its accreditation cycle and continues to meet the evolving needs of students, faculty, and the healthcare system. Internal review processes also foster a culture of continuous improvement, making it possible to identify areas of weakness, address them proactively, and ensure the program's long-term success.

Developing a Comprehensive Internal Review Framework

The internal review process should be comprehensive and include quantitative data collection and qualitative feedback. Data-driven decisions, supported by clear performance indicators, allow the program to assess student success, curriculum effectiveness, faculty performance, and overall program outcomes. By regularly reviewing this data, nursing programs can pinpoint areas for improvement and prioritize interventions accordingly.

A well-established internal review process is structured around several key elements, such as:

1. **Performance Metrics**: Key performance indicators (KPIs) such as NCLEX-RN pass rates, student retention, graduation rates, and employment outcomes are essential in monitoring a program's overall success. Tracking these metrics regularly allows program leaders to spot trends early on and take corrective action as needed.

2. **Student Feedback**: Students are one of the best sources of feedback regarding the quality of a nursing program. Their insights can highlight strengths and areas for improvement. This feedback can be collected through surveys, focus groups, or course evaluations. Topics of interest may include the effectiveness of instruction, the quality of clinical placements, and student satisfaction with academic support services.

3. **Faculty Assessments**: Faculty play a critical role in the success of a nursing program, so it's vital to assess their performance and professional development regularly. Faculty evaluations can include peer reviews, self-assessments, and student evaluations of teaching. This feedback helps identify professional development needs and ensures faculty maintain the expertise necessary to deliver high-quality education.

4. **Curriculum Reviews**: The curriculum should be regularly reviewed to align with accreditation standards and current industry practices. This process should involve faculty from different areas of expertise, clinical partners, and students to ensure the curriculum remains relevant and current. Faculty committees may meet semi-annually or annually to evaluate whether course content adequately prepares students for the clinical environment and meets the healthcare system's needs.

5. **Clinical Placement Evaluation**: Clinical placements are critical to nursing education, offering students practical experience in real-world healthcare settings. Regular evaluations of clinical sites and placements allow the program to ensure that students are getting adequate hands-on training. Feedback from clinical preceptors, nursing staff, and students can help the program identify opportunities to improve the quality of these placements. Partnerships with healthcare organizations should be continuously nurtured to ensure the sustainability and quality of clinical training opportunities.

Building an Effective Internal Review Committee

A dedicated internal review committee is central to the review process. This committee should comprise key stakeholders, including faculty members, administrators, and staff. Still, it may also involve clinical partners and student representatives. Having a diverse group ensures that all perspectives are considered and that the review process is thorough.

The role of the internal review committee includes:

- Collecting and analyzing data related to the program's performance and identifying areas where the program excels and improvements are needed.
- Establish goals for continuous improvement and ensure that these goals align with accreditation standards.
- Collaborating with faculty and other stakeholders to develop and implement action plans for addressing deficiencies and improving program quality.
- Monitoring progress toward achieving established goals, adjusting plans as necessary, and ensuring that the program meets or exceeds accreditation requirements.

Ensuring Timely Action on Identified Issues

Once gaps or deficiencies are identified through the internal review, swift action is essential to correct them. Developing an action plan to address deficiencies and areas for improvement is an important part of the internal review. Action plans should outline specific steps, responsible parties, timelines, and resources to address each issue.

For example, if an internal review identifies a decline in student retention or a decrease in NCLEX-RN pass rates, the action plan could include additional support services such as tutoring, mentoring, or faculty workshops to address the issue. Monitoring progress over time and adjusting the plan ensures that improvements are sustainable.

Additionally, programs should track their action plans and document any changes made. This documentation is crucial when preparing for future accreditation reviews, as it demonstrates that the program is actively addressing any identified weaknesses and is committed to continuous quality improvement.

Fostering a Culture of Continuous Improvement

A strong internal review process also fosters a culture of continuous improvement within the program. Faculty, staff, and administrators should view the review process not as a time-consuming bureaucratic task but as an opportunity to improve the program, refine teaching methods, enhance student learning experiences, and contribute to its success meeting accreditation standards.

Regularly reviewing and acting upon data-driven insights encourages a growth mindset where the program strives to improve. Faculty development programs, faculty research, curricular adjustments, and enhancements to student support services should all be part of this ongoing improvement process. By adopting continuous improvement as a core value, nursing programs ensure their long-term sustainability and the ability to adapt to changes in the healthcare environment.

The Role of Stakeholders in the Internal Review Process

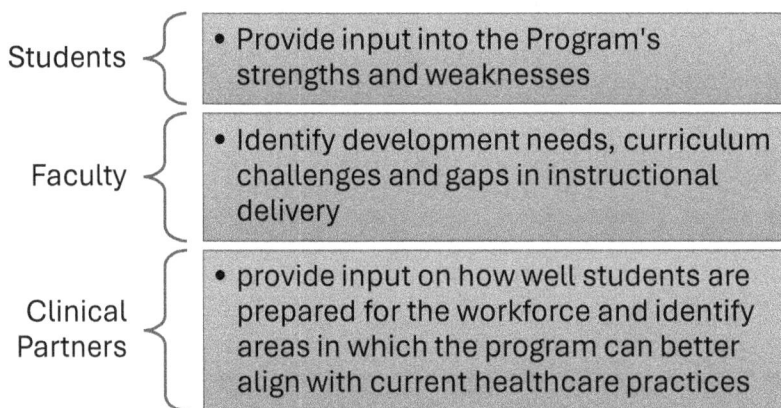

Students	• Provide input into the Program's strengths and weaknesses
Faculty	• Identify development needs, curriculum challenges and gaps in instructional delivery
Clinical Partners	• provide input on how well students are prepared for the workforce and identify areas in which the program can better align with current healthcare practices

Figure 10 The Role of Stakeholders in the Internal Review Process

Stakeholders, including students, faculty, staff, and clinical partners, should be engaged in the internal review process to gather a broad range of feedback. Students input on their educational experience provides critical insights into the program's strengths and weaknesses. At the same time, faculty feedback can identify professional development needs, curriculum challenges, and gaps in instructional delivery.

Clinical partners can provide input on how well students are prepared for the workforce and identify areas where the program can better align with current healthcare practices. Engaging clinical partners in the review process helps ensure that the program meets the needs of both students and employers.

A good practice for keeping stakeholders engaged is hosting regular meetings or surveys to solicit feedback. This information should be shared and discussed with faculty, who can make decisions and adjustments based on stakeholder input.

Conclusion

Establishing a robust internal review process for ongoing quality assurance is key to maintaining accreditation and ensuring the continued success of a nursing program. By systematically collecting data, involving all stakeholders, promptly addressing deficiencies, and committing to continuous improvement, programs can remain compliant with accreditation standards and continue to provide high-quality education to future nurses. This internal review process should be ingrained in the program's culture and considered an essential component of the program's long-term success.

7.2 Engaging Stakeholders in Continuous Self-Assessment and Program Development

A successful accreditation process is driven by the active engagement of all stakeholders involved in the nursing program. This includes faculty, students, clinical partners, administrators, and employers. All these groups provide essential feedback that can help identify areas of the program that need improvement or adaptation.

One of the most effective ways to engage stakeholders in self-assessment is through regular surveys, focus groups, and feedback mechanisms. For instance, student satisfaction surveys can offer insights into how well the program meets student needs regarding instruction, clinical placements, and academic support. Alumni surveys can provide feedback on how well the program prepared them for practice in the field.

Clinical partners also play a critical role in assessing the program's effectiveness, ensuring students receive adequate training in real-world healthcare environments. By engaging clinical partners in discussions about the program's strengths and weaknesses, nursing programs can identify areas where students might need additional training or experience.

Additionally, nursing programs should encourage open communication between faculty and administrators. Regular meetings can help align program goals with accreditation standards while ensuring faculty concerns and recommendations are heard and acted upon. Engaging faculty in these discussions fosters a culture of collaboration and continuous improvement, ensuring that the program remains responsive to the needs of both students and the healthcare community.

7.3 Keeping Up with Changing Accreditation Standards and Expectations

Accreditation standards are not static, and nursing programs must stay informed about these standards changes. Accrediting agencies often update their guidelines to reflect changes in the healthcare system, technological advancements, or shifts in educational best practices. Failure to stay current with these changes could result in the program failing to comply with accreditation standards, jeopardizing its accredited status.

Staying informed about changes in accreditation standards requires active participation in professional organizations and regular communication with accrediting bodies. Programs can subscribe to newsletters and publications from organizations like the *Commission on Collegiate Nursing Education* (CCNE) or the *Accreditation Commission for Education in Nursing* (ACEN), which often provide updates about changes in policies and standards.

Additionally, attending conferences and workshops hosted by accrediting agencies or professional nursing organizations can provide program leaders with opportunities to learn about emerging trends and standards in nursing education. This ongoing professional development ensures that the program is always prepared for changes in accreditation requirements.

Case Study
Examples of Programs That Excel at Maintaining Accreditation
Case Study 1: Urban University Nursing Program An urban nursing program in a large metropolitan area achieved accreditation and maintained it successfully by establishing a comprehensive system for continuous improvement. The program implemented a quality assurance committee of faculty, administrators, and clinical

partners. This committee met quarterly to review performance data, identify potential gaps in the curriculum, and ensure alignment with accreditation standards. As a result, the program maintained its accreditation status and received commendations for its strong focus on student outcomes, particularly regarding NCLEX-RN pass and employment rates for graduates.

Case Study 2: Rural Nursing Program A rural nursing program faced unique challenges due to limited resources and geographic isolation. However, the program maintained its accreditation by forming strong partnerships with local healthcare organizations. These partnerships provided valuable clinical placements for students and offered resources for faculty development. The program's commitment to continuous self-assessment and an innovative approach to clinical training enabled it to meet accreditation standards and achieve excellent graduate employment outcomes in underserved areas.

Summary

Maintaining accreditation post-approval requires a dynamic and proactive approach. Nursing programs can maintain their accredited status by staying on top of accreditation timelines, preparing for periodic reports, developing systems for continuous quality improvement, and engaging stakeholders. With ongoing self-assessment and adaptation to changes in accreditation standards, programs can continue to provide high-quality education that meets the needs of students, healthcare organizations, and the broader healthcare system.

Key terms for Chapter 7

1. **Periodic Reports**
   Regular reports submitted by accredited programs to demonstrate ongoing compliance with accreditation standards between full accreditation reviews.

2. **Reaccreditation**
   The process through which a nursing program must undergo periodic evaluation and reassessment to maintain its accredited status, typically occurring every 5–10 years.

3. **Continuous Quality Improvement (CQI)**
   An ongoing effort to improve processes, systems, and outcomes to enhance the nursing program's overall quality.

4. **Internal Review Process**
   The method by which a nursing program internally evaluates its compliance with accreditation standards monitors performance, and makes improvements.

5. **Feedback and Recommendations**
   Input from accrediting bodies or external evaluators regarding the program's performance, including suggestions for improvement or areas requiring attention.

6. **Action Plan**
   A detailed strategy developed by the nursing program to address deficiencies or recommendations from accreditation feedback, aimed at improving quality.

7. **Data Collection**
   The systematic gathering of quantitative and qualitative data related to program performance, student outcomes, and faculty effectiveness.

8. **Performance Metrics**
   Key indicators such as student retention rates, NCLEX-RN pass rates, graduation rates, and employment outcomes are used to measure the success of the nursing program.

9. **Program Development**
   Refine and enhance the nursing program to meet better accreditation standards, student needs, and healthcare industry requirements.

10. **Program Evaluation**
    The process of assessing the effectiveness and outcomes of a nursing program concerning its goals and accreditation standards.

11. **Quality Assurance**
    A systematic process of monitoring and improving the quality of educational services, curriculum, and student outcomes to ensure continued accreditation.

12. **Stakeholder Engagement** –
    The active participation of various individuals and groups (e.g., faculty, students, clinical partners) in the process of evaluating and improving the nursing program.

End of Chapter Questions:

Multiple Choice Questions

1. Which of the following is NOT a typical step in the reaccreditation process for nursing programs?
   A. Submission of periodic reports
   B. Complete re-evaluation of program faculty
   C. Self-study and external review
   D. Continuous monitoring of program outcomes
2. The primary purpose of an internal review process in maintaining accreditation is to:
   A. Ensure compliance with local regulations
   B. Identify areas for program improvement
   C. Increase the program's student enrollment
   D. Promote faculty development programs
3. How often do most nursing programs undergo reaccreditation reviews?
   A. Every 1-2 years

   B. Every 3-5 years
   C. Every 5-10 years
   D. Every 15-20 years
4. Which of the following is essential for a nursing program to maintain its accreditation status?
   A. Regular updates to the program's website
   B. Submission of periodic reports that show ongoing compliance
   C. Offering at least ten clinical placements annually
   D. Implementing faculty sabbaticals every 5 years
5. What is one key advantage of engaging stakeholders in continuous self-assessment and program development?
   A. Reduces the cost of the program
   B. Enhances alignment with healthcare industry needs
   C. Increases student retention rates to 100%
   D. Allows faculty to pursue research projects freely

True/False Questions

6. The reaccreditation process is typically conducted by the same agency that initially accredited the program.
   True / False
7. Periodic reports submitted during reaccreditation cycles focus mainly on the financial health of the nursing program.
   True / False
8. Stakeholders, such as faculty and students, play no significant role in the ongoing accreditation process after initial approval.
   True / False
9. The internal review process is only conducted in the year immediately before reaccreditation.
   True / False
10. A nursing program's ability to meet ongoing accreditation standards largely depends on continuous quality improvement and data-driven decisions.
    True / False

Short Answer Questions

11. What is the primary role of periodic reports in maintaining accreditation for nursing programs?
12. How does an internal review process contribute to continuous quality improvement in nursing programs?
13. Why is it important to involve key stakeholders, such as faculty and students, in the accreditation maintenance process?
14. What are some common challenges nursing programs face in maintaining accreditation, and how can these be addressed?
15. Describe the relationship between keeping up with changing accreditation standards and the ongoing success of a nursing program.

Essay Questions

16. Explain the key components of a successful internal review process for maintaining accreditation. In your response, discuss how data collection, stakeholder feedback, and faculty involvement contribute to the effectiveness of the review.
17. Discuss the steps a nursing program should take to prepare for reaccreditation. Include how the program can use previous feedback and data to demonstrate continuous improvement.
18. How can nursing programs maintain continuous quality improvement between accreditation cycles? Explore how ongoing assessment, the use of technology, and stakeholder engagement play key roles in this process.

Chapter 8
Addressing Challenges in the Accreditation Journey

Accreditation ensures that nursing programs meet the highest education standards, quality, and relevance in healthcare. While the benefits of accreditation are clear—such as improved program quality, enhanced reputation, and increased funding opportunities—nursing programs often face significant challenges throughout the accreditation journey. These challenges can arise from various factors, including financial limitations, staffing shortages, changes in leadership, and shifts in external regulations. How well a program navigates these obstacles can make the difference between maintaining or losing accreditation altogether.

This chapter examines the common barriers nursing programs face during accreditation and how to address them. It also provides strategies for enhancing program resilience, managing change effectively, and ensuring continuous improvement to stay aligned with evolving accreditation requirements.

8.1 Overcoming Common Barriers: Financial Constraints, Staffing Shortages, and Resource Limitations

Financial constraints, staffing shortages, and resource limitations are significant barriers that nursing programs must address to achieve and maintain accreditation. These obstacles can directly impact a program's ability to meet the rigorous standards established by accrediting bodies like the *Accreditation Commission for Education in Nursing* (ACEN) or the *Commission on Collegiate Nursing Education* (CCNE).

Financial Constraints

Nursing programs often face challenges in securing adequate funding to support the various elements of accreditation, including faculty recruitment and retention, technology investments, clinical placement opportunities, and student services. This is particularly true for public institutions, smaller schools, and programs located in underserved or rural areas. According to a 2021 *American Association of Colleges of Nursing* (AACN) survey, about 30% of nursing programs reported significant financial constraints that hindered their ability to maintain or enhance accreditation standards.

However, some strategies can help overcome financial limitations. Creative partnerships with healthcare organizations, government grants, and alumni donations can help nursing programs increase their funding. Partnerships with local hospitals or clinics, for instance, not only allow nursing programs to provide valuable clinical placements for students but can also secure funding to improve faculty development or enhance simulation labs, all of which are important for meeting accreditation standards.

Staffing Shortages

Staffing shortages, especially among nursing faculty, are another persistent challenge. The *National League for Nursing* (NLN) reports that more than 1,000 nursing programs have had to leave faculty positions unfilled due to the ongoing shortage of qualified nursing educators. Staffing challenges can result in a program being unable to meet accreditation standards for faculty-student ratios, faculty qualifications, and professional development requirements.

To overcome staffing shortages, programs must focus on recruitment and retention strategies. Offering competitive salaries, benefits, and professional development opportunities, such as faculty mentoring and research grants, can help attract and retain qualified educators. Additionally, creating flexible teaching roles, including part-time or adjunct faculty positions, can alleviate the pressure on full-time staff and ensure that the program meets accreditation expectations. Moreover, fostering strong partnerships with local healthcare systems can provide access to experienced clinicians who can teach part-time, thus alleviating the burden on the core faculty.

Resource Limitations

Limited equipment, facilities, and technology resources can significantly hinder accreditation for many nursing programs. Accrediting bodies require that nursing programs have adequate clinical spaces, laboratories, and access to technology to train students effectively. However, the *National Council of State Boards of Nursing* (NCSBN) has noted that some nursing programs struggle with outdated or insufficient resources, which makes it challenging to provide students with the hands-on experience necessary for clinical competency.

One-way programs can address resource limitations by leveraging simulation technology. Simulations allow students to practice clinical skills in a controlled environment, making them a valuable tool for nursing education. Many nursing programs have incorporated high-fidelity simulation labs to meet accreditation requirements for clinical experiences, even with limited opportunities for in-person clinical placements. Simulation offers students real-world practice and allows programs to better manage resource constraints without compromising educational quality.

8.2 Dealing with Non-Compliance or Failure to Meet Accreditation Standards

Occasionally, nursing programs may face situations that do not meet the accreditation standards of agencies like ACEN or CCNE. This could occur for various reasons, such as low NCLEX-RN pass rates, inadequate faculty qualifications, or failure to meet student outcome goals. While non-compliance can be concerning, it is important to understand that it is not an insurmountable obstacle. Programs can take corrective actions and work closely with accrediting bodies to address deficiencies and get back on track.

Identifying Areas of Non-Compliance

When a program receives feedback that it does not comply with certain accreditation standards, it is crucial to review the areas of concern carefully. These might include academic quality, faculty development, clinical experiences, or student outcomes. For example, a nursing program that experiences a dip in NCLEX-RN pass rates may need to reassess its curriculum, provide additional remediation support, or increase faculty engagement in preparing students for licensure exams.

Developing a Corrective Action Plan

Once areas of non-compliance are identified, programs must develop a corrective action plan to address them. This plan should include clear, actionable steps with defined timelines and measurable outcomes. For example, a program that struggles with low faculty qualifications might implement a professional development program to help instructors meet the necessary academic credentials. Similarly, a program that fails to meet student retention goals might create an early intervention system to support at-risk students and improve retention rates.

Engaging with Accrediting Bodies

Maintaining open communication with the accrediting body during the corrective action process is also essential. Accrediting agencies generally support programs that demonstrate a genuine commitment to improvement. By keeping the lines of communication open and providing evidence of the steps to address deficiencies, nursing programs can rebuild trust and successfully regain full accreditation status.

8.3 Navigating Changes in Leadership or Faculty During the Accreditation Process

Leadership changes can significantly affect the accreditation process. A new program director or dean may bring a different vision or set of priorities, which can alter the direction of the program's accreditation journey. Similarly, faculty turnover can disrupt continuity in teaching, curriculum delivery, and clinical supervision. Both leadership and faculty changes can impact the program's ability to meet accreditation standards. They may even result in delays or complications during site visits.

Ensuring Continuity Through Leadership Transitions

To ensure continuity, nursing programs should establish a succession planning process, which includes training and preparing potential leaders well before a transition. This allows new leadership to step into their roles with a clear understanding of the accreditation process and the program's goals. Additionally, involving key faculty members in the accreditation process ensures that their expertise and commitment remain integral to the program's success, regardless of leadership changes.

Managing Faculty Transitions

Similarly, faculty turnover can be minimized by creating a strong faculty development and mentorship culture. By offering ongoing training opportunities, faculty members can continue to grow professionally while meeting the qualifications required by accreditation agencies. Furthermore, programs can create mentorship networks for new faculty members, which can help them acclimate to the program's expectations and ensure consistent delivery of high-quality education.

8.4 Handling External Challenges: Changes in Regulations, Healthcare Trends

Accreditation standards are not static; they evolve in response to changes in healthcare regulations, workforce demands, and emerging healthcare trends. For example, the widespread adoption of telehealth and other digital health technologies has prompted accrediting bodies to incorporate these topics into their standards. Nursing programs must adapt to these external challenges and ensure their curricula remain current and relevant to the changing healthcare environment.

Adapting to Regulatory Changes

Changes in healthcare regulations or workforce needs can also impact a program's ability to maintain accreditation. Nursing programs must stay informed about changes in state licensure requirements, clinical practice standards, and national healthcare policies. Regularly reviewing relevant regulations, engaging in professional development activities, and participating in healthcare policy discussions can help nursing programs remain proactive in meeting evolving accreditation standards.

Responding to Healthcare Trends

In addition to regulatory changes, emerging healthcare trends—such as the growing emphasis on interprofessional collaboration, patient-centered care, and diversity in healthcare—may require nursing programs to adjust curricula. Programs should actively seek partnerships with healthcare providers to ensure that their curriculum reflects real-world practices and that students are prepared for the current healthcare landscape.

8.5 Strategies for Program Resilience and Adaptability

Resilience and adaptability are crucial for nursing programs that aim to maintain accreditation and thrive despite external challenges. Programs must respond with agility and foresight to financial constraints, staffing shortages, regulatory shifts, and faculty changes.

Building a Culture of Continuous Improvement

A key strategy for resilience is fostering a culture of continuous improvement within the program. This involves consistently gathering data on student performance, faculty effectiveness, and program outcomes and using that data to make informed decisions about how to improve. A program that emphasizes feedback, self-assessment, and stakeholder engagement is more likely to adapt successfully to changes and overcome obstacles.

Engaging Stakeholders in Program Development

Finally, engaging all key stakeholders—faculty, students, administrators, and healthcare partners—through regular communication and collaboration can strengthen the program's adaptability. Involving stakeholders in decision-making processes ensures that the program remains relevant, responsive, and prepared to meet the evolving needs of students and the healthcare system.

Key terms for Chapter 8

1. **Accreditation Barriers**
   Obstacles that programs face when trying to meet accreditation standards including financial, staffing, and resource limitations.

2. **Non-Compliance**
   Failure to meet the established accreditation standards may result in a program being placed on probation or losing accreditation status.

3. **Corrective Action Plan**
   A strategy developed by a program in response to non-compliance outlines the steps to meet the required standards.

4. **Faculty Turnover**
   The rate at which faculty leave a program can disrupt continuity in teaching and curriculum development, affecting accreditation outcomes.

5. **Leadership Changes**
   Transition or turnover in leadership, such as the program director or dean, can impact the accreditation process's stability and direction.

6. **Regulatory Changes**
   Modifications to laws, policies, or accreditation standards that programs must adapt to maintain compliance and accreditation status.

7. **Healthcare Trends**
   Nursing programs must incorporate shifting dynamics in the healthcare industry, such as the rise of telehealth, to remain relevant and meet accreditation standards.

8. **Program Resilience**
   The ability of a nursing program to adapt to challenges and changes while maintaining the quality of education and fulfilling accreditation requirements.

9. **Continuous Improvement**
   Ongoing efforts to enhance the quality of the program, based on assessment data, feedback, and evolving accreditation standards.

10. **Stakeholder Engagement**

Involving faculty, staff, students, and external partners in the accreditation process, ensuring that all relevant parties are invested in achieving and maintaining accreditation.

End of Chapter Questions

1. What are some of the most common barriers nursing programs face when pursuing accreditation?

2. How can a program effectively respond to non-compliance with accreditation standards?

3. Why is faculty turnover a significant challenge in the accreditation process, and what strategies can programs use to minimize its impact?

4. Explain the potential consequences of leadership changes during the accreditation process and suggest effective ways to manage these transitions.

5. What are some external challenges nursing programs may encounter that could impact their ability to meet accreditation standards?

6. What steps can a nursing program take to build resilience and adaptability in the face of accreditation challenges?

7. How can a program's leadership foster continuous improvement to ensure the long-term success of the accreditation process?

8. Discuss how a corrective action plan can be used to address areas of non-compliance in a nursing program.

9. What role does stakeholder engagement play in maintaining accreditation, and how can programs ensure that all relevant parties are actively involved in the accreditation process?

10. How can nursing programs navigate healthcare trends and regulatory updates while maintaining accreditation standards?

Chapter 9
The Role of Accreditation in Advancing Nursing Education

9.1 How Accreditation Affects the Nursing Profession

Accreditation is an essential aspect of nursing education, significantly shaping the quality of care provided within the healthcare system. It is a mechanism that guarantees nursing programs adhere to national standards of educational excellence, ensuring that graduates are equipped with the necessary skills and knowledge to meet the demands of the healthcare field. The process involves a thorough evaluation by accrediting bodies such as the *Accreditation Commission for Education in Nursing* (ACEN) and the *Commission on Collegiate Nursing Education* (CCNE), which assess a variety of factors, including curriculum, faculty qualifications, clinical placements, and overall program effectiveness.

The importance of accreditation cannot be overstated. A well-established accreditation system maintains the integrity of nursing education. It ensures that nursing programs remain aligned with contemporary healthcare needs. Accreditation drives the continuous improvement of educational standards, encouraging institutions to stay current with advancements in medical technology, nursing practices, and healthcare policy. Integrating the latest evidence-based practices into nursing curricula enhances the competency of graduates, which directly benefits patient care.

The research underscores the positive impact of accreditation on the nursing profession. According to the *American Association of Colleges of Nursing* (AACN), 94% of registered nurses (RNs) in the U.S. graduate from accredited programs. Accreditation guarantees that the educational process meets rigorous standards, thus preparing a highly competent workforce. It also reassures employers and patients that nurses have the appropriate knowledge and clinical skills to deliver safe and effective care. This is critical as the demand for quality healthcare continues to rise in a world facing aging populations, increasing rates of chronic diseases, and the constant evolution of medical technology.

Impact on Students: Employment Opportunities, Licensure, and Career Advancement

Accreditation influences the educational quality of nursing programs and directly impacts students' professional prospects. The credibility that comes with graduating from an accredited nursing program is vital for securing employment. Employers often prefer accredited programs, as they offer assurance that graduates have received the necessary education to deliver high-quality care in a clinical setting. This enhances employability for nursing students, with graduates from accredited programs typically experiencing higher job placement rates and quicker employment post-graduation.

For instance, a 2021 survey by the AACN found that graduates from accredited nursing programs had a 95% employment rate within six months of obtaining their licensure. In contrast, non-accredited programs often result in lower employment outcomes. This can be attributed to the superior education and training in accredited programs, which better prepare students for the challenges they will face in healthcare settings. In addition, accredited nursing programs are more likely to have clinical partnerships with hospitals and healthcare organizations, which provides students with valuable hands-on experience.

Moreover, accreditation ensures that nursing students are eligible to sit for the *National Council Licensure Examination for Registered Nurses* (NCLEX-RN), a requirement for licensure in the U.S. Many states mandate that only graduates of accredited nursing programs are eligible to take the exam, which reinforces the importance of accreditation in the licensure process. Passing the NCLEX-RN is essential for nurses to practice legally, and graduating from an accredited program is critical to achieving licensure and advancing in one's nursing career.

Accreditation also affects long-term career development. Nurses trained in accredited programs tend to pursue higher education opportunities, such as advanced practice roles, specialty certifications, and doctoral programs. A National Nursing Workforce Survey study showed that nurses with a BSN from an accredited program are more likely to pursue advanced practice roles, such as nurse practitioner, clinical nurse specialist, or nurse educator. These roles offer higher salaries, increased job satisfaction, and more significant influence within healthcare teams.

Enhancing Public Trust and Confidence in Nursing Programs

Accreditation is crucial in building and maintaining public trust in nursing education programs. In an era where patients are becoming more informed and involved in their healthcare decisions, ensuring that nurses are adequately educated is the key to fostering trust within the healthcare system. Accreditation provides external validation that a nursing program meets high standards of educational quality and produces graduates who are well-prepared for clinical practice.

The transparency of the accreditation process allows the public to have confidence that nursing programs are subject to rigorous evaluation. Accreditation agencies conduct thorough assessments of a program's curriculum, faculty qualifications, clinical training sites, and outcomes, ensuring that each aspect of the program meets or exceeds established standards. This accountability reassures patients and their families that the nurses are highly trained and competent.

Public trust is essential for the overall effectiveness of the healthcare system, and accreditation ensures that nursing programs contribute positively to this trust. The *National Nursing Workforce Survey* found that 84% of healthcare leaders consider accreditation essential when choosing educational programs for clinical placements or hiring decisions. This statistic highlights how accreditation strengthens the credibility of nursing programs and reinforces the public's confidence in the nursing profession.

Collaboration with Healthcare Institutions to Improve Clinical Placements and Outcomes

One of the most significant benefits of accreditation is the collaboration between nursing programs and healthcare institutions. Clinical placements, where nursing students gain hands-on experience, are a critical part of the nursing education process. Accredited programs are likelier to have established partnerships with hospitals, clinics, and other healthcare organizations, providing students with opportunities to learn in diverse and dynamic environments.

These partnerships allow nursing students to practice their clinical skills under the supervision of experienced professionals, bridging the gap between theoretical knowledge and practical application. Furthermore, accredited programs often work closely with healthcare institutions to improve clinical training, ensuring students are exposed to the latest healthcare practices and technologies. This collaboration not only enhances the student's education but also contributes to improved patient care outcomes.

According to the Journal of Nursing Education, nursing programs collaborating with healthcare institutions report better clinical placement opportunities for students and improved performance on the NCLEX-RN exam. In addition, these partnerships often result in improved retention rates for students and healthcare employees, as students with a favorable clinical placement experience are more likely to seek employment with the institutions they trained at. This mutual benefit is one of the key advantages of accreditation, as it strengthens the relationship between educational institutions and healthcare providers.

9.2 Future Trends in Nursing Education Accreditation and Its Evolving Role

As healthcare continues to evolve, so must the accreditation process for nursing programs. Several emerging trends, reflecting the changing needs of the healthcare system and the nursing profession, are likely to shape the future of nursing education accreditation.

One significant trend is the increasing focus on interprofessional education (IPE), which encourages collaboration between nursing students and students from other healthcare disciplines, such as medicine, pharmacy, and social work. Accrediting bodies are beginning to emphasize the importance of IPE in improving patient care. They are incorporating these requirements into accreditation standards. Research has shown that interprofessional collaboration improves patient outcomes, reduces healthcare costs, and enhances the quality of care. Therefore, nursing programs must focus on preparing students to work effectively in multidisciplinary healthcare teams.

Another trend is the incorporation of technology into nursing education. As healthcare becomes more digitized, nurses must be equipped with the skills to navigate electronic health records, telemedicine platforms, and other digital health tools. Accrediting agencies emphasize integrating technology into nursing curricula to ensure that students are prepared for the technological demands of modern healthcare environments.

The issue of nursing faculty shortages will also continue to shape the future of nursing education accreditation. The AACN reports that nearly 70,000 qualified applicants were turned away from nursing programs in 2020 due to faculty shortages. To address this challenge, accreditation agencies may revise standards to focus more on faculty development, recruitment, and retention strategies. This could include developing programs to enhance faculty training and providing incentives for experienced clinicians to enter the field of nursing education.

Lastly, lifelong learning will become an even more integral part of nursing education and accreditation. As healthcare knowledge rapidly evolves, there will be an increased focus on ensuring that nursing programs prepare students for entry-level practice and foster an environment that encourages ongoing professional development. This will require nursing programs to integrate continuous education opportunities into their curricula and support nurses pursuing advanced degrees and certifications.

Key terms for Chapter 9

1. **Global Health Workforce**
   The international network of health professionals, including nurses, whose skills and training are essential in addressing global healthcare needs, particularly in underserved regions.

End of Chapter Questions

1. What is the role of accreditation in nursing education, and why is it important for nursing programs?
2. How does accreditation impact employment opportunities for nursing graduates?
3. Explain the relationship between accreditation and licensure for nursing students.
4. In what ways does accreditation enhance public trust and confidence in nursing programs?
5. How can nursing programs collaborate with healthcare institutions to improve student clinical placements and outcomes?
6. What are future trends in nursing education accreditation, and how might they impact the profession?
7. How do accreditation standards affect the development of nursing curricula and the quality of education provided?
8. Describe the impact of accredited nursing programs on the healthcare workforce and patient care outcomes.
9. What are the potential consequences for a nursing program if it fails to maintain accreditation?
10. Why is program evaluation critical for maintaining accreditation, and how does it contribute to continuous improvement?

Chapter 10
Special Accreditations

Nursing education is diverse, encompassing a range of specialized fields that cater to the dynamic needs of healthcare. While general nursing education accreditation ensures a foundational level of quality, some nursing disciplines require specialized accreditation due to their complexity and scope. This chapter focuses on two critical areas of special accreditation: Simulation Program Accreditation and Nurse Anesthesia Program Accreditation, highlighting their unique standards, the processes involved, and their impact on nursing education and healthcare delivery.

10.1 Simulation Program Accreditation

Simulation-based learning has become an indispensable tool in modern nursing education. Through simulations, nursing students can practice and hone their clinical skills in a safe, controlled environment, preparing them for real-life scenarios without risking patient safety. However, as the use of simulation continues to grow, the need for formal accreditation has risen to ensure these programs meet high educational quality and safety standards.

Importance of Simulation Accreditation

Accrediting simulation programs is crucial for providing effective learning experiences that meet educational and patient safety standards. The *Society for Simulation in Healthcare* (SSH) is one of the leading accrediting bodies for simulation programs, offering a comprehensive accreditation process for programs that integrate simulation into their curricula. The SSH standards ensure that simulation programs are well-structured, evidence-based, and effective in achieving measurable learning outcomes.

To be accredited by SSH, a simulation program must demonstrate several key features:

- **Integration with Clinical Education**: The program must show how simulations complement traditional clinical education and improve students' overall competency. This requires alignment with national nursing competency frameworks and clinical guidelines.

- **Faculty Expertise**: Instructors must have specific training and experience in simulation-based education. They should also be knowledgeable in debriefing techniques, which are critical to the reflection and learning that occurs post-simulation.

- **Assessment and Evaluation**: Accreditation requires that simulation programs implement robust mechanisms for assessing student performance during the simulation and post-simulation debriefing. Programs must provide objective criteria for evaluating student performance in simulated clinical scenarios.

- **Student Engagement and Learning Outcomes**: Evidence must be documented that simulation activities effectively engage students and contribute to their clinical decision-making, teamwork, and leadership skills. Accreditation requires programs to provide outcome data such as student satisfaction, skill acquisition, and clinical performance improvements.

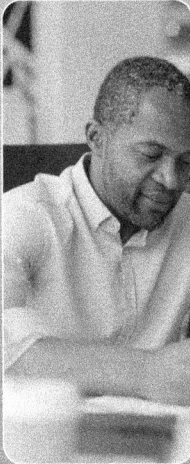

Society for Simulation in Healthcare

- **CORE**
  - **Standard 1** Mission & Governance
  - **Standard 2** Program Management
  - **Standard 3** Resource Management
  - **Standard 4** Human Resources
  - **Standard 5** Program Improvement
  - **Standard 6** Ethics
  - **Standard 7** Expanding the Field
- **TEACHING & EDUCATION**
  - **Standard 1** Teaching Activities
  - **Standard 2** Educational Activity Design
  - **Standard 3** Qualified Educators
  - **Standard 4** Evaluation & Improvement

Figure 11 SSH Core and Teaching Standards.
Note: SSH does offer additional accreditation in other areas as well: Assessment, Research, Systems Integration, and Fellowship

The Role of Simulation in Enhancing Clinical Skills

The use of simulation as a teaching tool has been shown to improve a variety of clinical skills. A study published in *Simulation in Healthcare* found that nursing students who participated in high-fidelity simulation-based learning scored significantly higher on clinical skill assessments, demonstrating better critical thinking, teamwork, and technical proficiency. The simulation environments allow students to experience various clinical situations—such as managing cardiac arrest, handling obstetrical emergencies, and practicing complex pharmacological interventions—that may not occur frequently during traditional clinical rotations.

A *National League for Nursing* (NLN) study revealed that programs utilizing accredited simulation curricula reported an 18% increase in student competency in high-stakes clinical situations, such as critical care management, compared to programs without simulation integration.

Benefits of Simulation Accreditation

Accredited simulation programs lead to better-prepared graduates who can immediately contribute to patient care upon entering the workforce. Using realistic, evidence-based scenarios allows students to refine their clinical judgment, communication, and leadership skills. Accreditation also provides a mark of quality for healthcare employers, who can be confident that nurses trained in accredited programs have mastered the necessary clinical competencies.

Moreover, simulation accreditation ensures the program's sustainability by fostering ongoing quality improvement. Accredited programs are periodically reviewed to assess the continued effectiveness of their teaching methods, the relevance of their scenarios, and the fidelity of their simulation environments, which results in the continuous evolution of the curriculum.

10.2 Nurse Anesthesia Program Accreditation

Nurse anesthesia is a specialized advanced nursing practice area requiring extensive clinical and academic preparation. Nurse anesthetists (CRNAs) administer anesthesia during surgeries, labor, and other medical procedures, and they play a vital role in ensuring patient safety in high-risk situations. Due to the critical nature of the work, Nurse Anesthesia Programs are held to stringent accreditation standards to ensure the competency and safety of graduates.

COA Accreditation for Nurse Anesthesia Programs

The *Council on Accreditation of Nurse Anesthesia Educational Programs* (COA) accredits nurse anesthesia programs across the United States. COA sets the standards for educational quality, clinical training, and faculty qualifications to ensure that CRNAs are equipped with the knowledge and skills needed to provide safe, effective anesthesia care. The COA's accreditation process involves a thorough evaluation of the program's:

- **Curriculum**: Nurse anesthesia programs must provide a rigorous curriculum that includes courses on advanced pharmacology, anesthetic techniques, pathophysiology, and anesthesia-related ethics. The curriculum must be designed to ensure that students are competent in administering anesthesia safely and managing patients under anesthesia.
- **Clinical Training**: Accreditation standards require that students complete a minimum number of clinical hours under direct supervision. Clinical training must involve a wide variety of anesthesia cases, including general, regional, and local anesthesia, as well as for special populations such as pediatric, geriatric, and critically ill patients.
- **Faculty Qualifications**: Faculty members in nurse anesthesia programs must hold advanced degrees in anesthesia or a related field and have substantial experience as practicing CRNAs. Faculty must engage in professional development activities, such as research, continuing education, and clinical practice, to remain current with advancements in the field.
- **Program Evaluation**: Nurse anesthesia programs must systematically evaluate their outcomes, including graduation rates, certification exam pass rates, and employment rates for graduates. This ensures that the program meets its educational goals and that students are prepared to enter the workforce as skilled professionals.

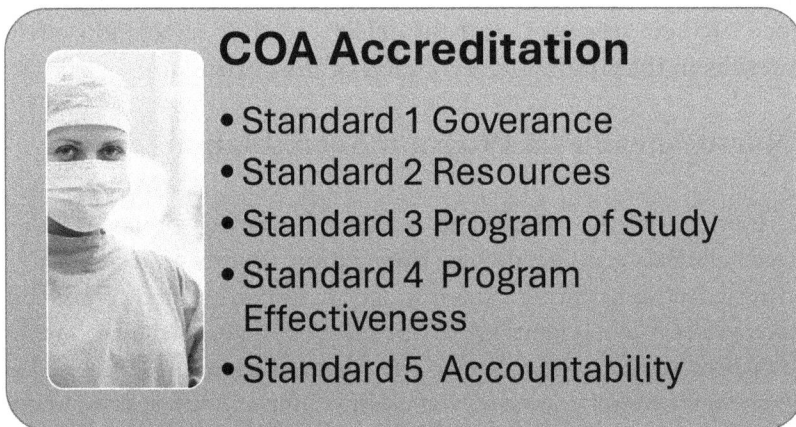

Figure 12 COA Accreditation Standards

Impact of Accreditation on Nurse Anesthesia Education

COA-accredited programs are widely recognized for producing highly competent CRNAs. Without accreditation, graduates would be ineligible to sit for the certification exam administered by the *National Board of Certification and*

Recertification for Nurse Anesthetists (NBCRNA). This would limit their ability to practice as CRNAs, significantly impacting their career prospects.

Studies have shown that CRNAs from COA-accredited programs report higher job satisfaction and are more likely to be employed in desirable clinical settings. The consistency and reliability of the education provided by accredited programs also ensure that nurse anesthetists meet the highest standards of patient care. A study in the *Journal of Clinical Anesthesia* found that hospitals with more CRNAs from accredited programs had lower complication rates during surgeries requiring anesthesia, suggesting that the quality of education directly impacts patient safety outcomes.

Trends in Nurse Anesthesia Education

One notable trend in nurse anesthesia education is the increasing adoption of simulation technology in training. With advancements in high-fidelity simulation mannequins and virtual reality, nurse anesthesia programs are incorporating simulation to allow students to practice anesthesia administration and patient monitoring in realistic, controlled settings. COA standards are evolving to include simulation as part of the educational experience, which enhances student competency and prepares them for real-world clinical challenges.

Another trend is the growing demand for nurse anesthesia educators. As the number of CRNA programs increases to meet the rising demand for anesthesia services, more advanced training programs for nurse anesthesia educators are being developed. This trend underscores the importance of maintaining high quality and teaching standards in these programs, ensuring the next generation of CRNAs is well-prepared.

Conclusion

Special accreditations, such as those for simulation and nurse anesthesia programs, are essential for ensuring that nursing education remains of the highest quality. These accreditations help maintain rigorous standards that benefit students, faculty, and patients alike. By focusing on evidence-based practices, clinical training, faculty development, and continuous improvement, accreditation provides an important framework for ensuring that nursing professionals are equipped to meet the evolving healthcare industry demands. As nursing education continues to evolve, these specialized accreditations will play a vital role in fostering the competency and success of the nursing workforce.

Key terms for Chapter 10

1. **Debriefing**:
   The process that follows a simulation exercise where students and instructors reflect on the activity, discussing what went well and areas for improvement. This is a critical component of simulation-based learning.

2. **Society for Simulation in Healthcare (SSH)**:
   A leading organization that accredits healthcare simulation programs, including nursing. SSH sets standards for quality and effectiveness in simulation-based learning.

3. **Council on Accreditation of Nurse Anesthesia Educational Programs (COA)**:
   The accrediting body for nurse anesthesia programs in the United States ensures these programs meet strict academic and clinical training standards.

4. **Clinical Training**:
   The hands-on component of nursing education is where students apply theoretical knowledge in a real-world healthcare setting under the supervision of experienced professionals.

5. **Certification Exam**:
   This is an examination that nursing graduates, particularly those in specialized fields like nurse anesthesia, must pass to become licensed to practice. For nurse anesthetists, this exam is administered by the National Board of Certification and Recertification for Nurse Anesthetists (NBCRNA).

6. **Nurse Anesthesia Program**:
   This specialized graduate program prepares registered nurses to become certified anesthetists (CRNAs). These programs require advanced education and clinical experience in anesthesia care.

7. **Clinical Competency**:
   The ability of a nursing student or nurse practitioner to perform tasks and make clinical decisions with a high degree of skill and accuracy is assessed through accreditation standards and ongoing evaluations.

8. **Accreditation Standards**:
   A set of criteria and expectations set by accrediting bodies to ensure that educational programs meet quality and safety standards. These standards often cover curriculum design, faculty qualifications, student outcomes, and clinical training.

9. **Outcome-Based Education**:
   This educational approach focuses on the learning process's results or outcomes, such as competency in clinical skills, critical thinking, and patient care.

10. **Simulation-Based Learning**:
    An instructional strategy that uses simulated clinical scenarios to teach nursing students skills, clinical decision-making, and teamwork in a risk-free environment.

11. **Advanced Practice Registered Nurse (APRN)**:
    A category of nursing professionals with advanced degrees and certification in specific practice fields, such as nurse anesthetists, nurse practitioners, and nurse midwives.

12. **Simulation Fidelity**:
    The degree to which a simulation closely replicates real-world conditions. High-fidelity simulations provide more realistic experiences that better prepare students for clinical practice.

13. **National Board of Certification and Recertification for Nurse Anesthetists (NBCRNA)**:
    The organization is responsible for certifying and recertifying nurse anesthetists. Graduates of accredited nurse anesthesia programs are eligible to sit for the certification exam administered by the NBCRNA.

14. **Program Evaluation**:
    The process by which an educational program assesses the effectiveness of its curriculum, teaching methods, and student outcomes. This is a key component of maintaining accreditation and ensuring continuous improvement.

15. **Clinical Hours**:
    The number of hours spent in direct patient care during a nursing education program is critical for accreditation and licensure. Nurse anesthesia programs have strict clinical hour requirements to ensure competency in anesthesia care.

16. **Interprofessional Education**:
    An approach to teaching that encourages collaboration among students from different healthcare disciplines (e.g., nursing, medicine, pharmacy) to improve patient care and outcomes.

17. **Evidence-Based Practice**:
    Integrating the best available research evidence, clinical expertise, and patient preferences into decision-making and practice. This is emphasized in both simulation and clinical education to ensure that nursing care is based on current best practices.

Conclusion
Achieving and Maintaining Nursing School Accreditation

Accreditation is the cornerstone for establishing the quality and integrity of nursing programs, ensuring they meet rigorous standards that prepare nurses for the complexities of healthcare environments. Obtaining and maintaining accreditation involves critical steps, from understanding accreditation bodies and their requirements to preparing for site visits and addressing feedback. Each step demands careful planning, collaboration, and a commitment to continuous improvement.

Recap of Key Steps to Achieve and Maintain Nursing School Accreditation

Achieving and maintaining accreditation begins with the initial understanding of the accrediting agency and its standards. Whether seeking initial accreditation or reaccreditation, programs must first understand the specific guidelines of agencies such as the *Accreditation Commission for Education in Nursing* (ACEN) or the *Commission on Collegiate Nursing Education* (CCNE). Programs must align their mission, goals, and educational outcomes with these standards, ensuring they meet both the requirements for quality education and the expectations for workforce readiness.

The next crucial step in the accreditation journey is the self-study process. As outlined in previous chapters, this involves thoroughly evaluating the program's resources, faculty, curriculum, student outcomes, and facilities. A comprehensive self-study enables programs to identify areas of strength and areas needing improvement. The process must be well-organized, with evidence-based support for all claims made in the report. Faculty, administrators, and students must be engaged in this process to ensure their perspectives are accurately represented and considered.

After completing the self-study, the program must prepare for the site visit. The site visit is integral to the accreditation process, where external evaluators assess the program's compliance with accreditation standards. Preparation for the site visit involves organizing logistics, preparing faculty and students for interviews, and ensuring that all documentation is current. The site visitors will review the program's policies, speak with key stakeholders, and assess facilities. Programs that provide comprehensive documentation and demonstrate an ongoing commitment to meeting accreditation standards are more likely to succeed.

The accreditation process's final phase involves responding to the accrediting agency's feedback. This feedback often includes recommendations for improvements. Addressing these recommendations may require developing action plans, adjusting policies, or improving specific areas within the program. For example, improving faculty qualifications or enhancing student support services may be necessary to meet the standards outlined in the agency's feedback. A program's ability to adapt and respond to such feedback is vital to sustaining its accreditation status.

Once accreditation is granted, it's essential to recognize that it is not a one-time achievement but an ongoing commitment. Maintaining accreditation requires regular reporting, participation in reaccreditation cycles, and continuous internal reviews. Programs must develop systems for monitoring their outcomes, ensuring they comply with accreditation standards. This includes reviewing student retention rates, NCLEX pass rates, employment outcomes, and implementing continuous quality improvement strategies. As accreditation standards evolve, programs must stay informed about changes to remain compliant.

Final Thoughts on the Importance of Accreditation for the Success of Nursing Programs

Accreditation is a matter of meeting regulatory requirements and a vital tool for ensuring that nursing programs provide students with the highest education and training standards. Research has shown that accredited programs lead to higher licensure pass rates, better job placement outcomes, and improved student satisfaction. For example, nursing programs with accreditation have a higher NCLEX pass rate, directly influencing the program's reputation and the future of its graduates. According to the *National Council of State Boards of Nursing* (NCSBN), programs that maintain accreditation typically report an average NCLEX pass rate of 90% or higher, compared to lower rates among non-accredited programs.

Accreditation also provides programs with access to resources and guidance to foster innovation and growth. Accredited programs are more likely to receive funding and grants, as many governmental and private organizations require accreditation for eligibility. The positive impact of accreditation on program funding cannot be overstated, as it allows institutions to invest in faculty development, student resources, and clinical partnerships, all of which improve the overall quality of education. Furthermore, accreditation enhances a program's credibility, boosting public trust in nursing education and ensuring that nurses are well-prepared to meet the healthcare industry's challenges.

Accreditation assures students a quality education that employers and licensing bodies will recognize. Graduating from an accredited program also increases employability, as healthcare institutions often prioritize hiring graduates from accredited nursing schools. Moreover, aligning the program's curriculum with industry standards and national competencies helps ensure students are prepared for real-world practice, making them more competitive in the job market.

The value of a well-trained nursing workforce cannot be understated for healthcare systems. As the demand for healthcare services grows, particularly with aging populations and increasing healthcare needs, accredited nursing programs are crucial in addressing workforce shortages. By ensuring that nursing programs meet high education standards, accreditation ultimately helps improve the quality of care delivered in healthcare settings.

Call to Action: Preparing Your Nursing Program for a Successful Accreditation Journey

For nursing programs seeking accreditation or reaccreditation, it is crucial to recognize that the process requires significant effort, collaboration, and long-term commitment. By following the outlined steps and focusing on continuous improvement, programs can meet and exceed the accreditation standards, providing students with an educational experience that is second to none.

A proactive approach is essential for success. Program leaders should begin the process well in advance, establishing a clear plan that includes timelines, assigned responsibilities, and mechanisms for ongoing monitoring. Faculty and administrators must work closely to ensure that all aspects of the program meet accreditation standards. Fostering an environment of collaboration, where faculty, students, and staff are engaged in the self-study and feedback processes, can strengthen the program's ability to adapt to changes and continuously improve.

As accreditation standards evolve and the healthcare landscape changes, nursing programs must stay flexible and responsive. By prioritizing evidence-based practices, student success, and faculty development, programs can ensure that they meet accreditation requirements and position themselves as leaders in nursing education.

In conclusion, accreditation is critical to the growth and success of nursing programs. It is more than a regulatory requirement; it is an essential tool for ensuring that nursing education prepares the workforce to meet the needs of patients and healthcare systems in the years to come. Programs that embrace accreditation and view it as an ongoing journey rather than a one-time achievement will continue to thrive and contribute to advancing the nursing profession.

Appendix A.
Sources of Data to Evaluate Programs in Nursing

Introduction

Evaluating nursing programs effectively requires comprehensive data from diverse sources to assess student outcomes, faculty performance, curriculum effectiveness, and overall program quality. Below is a categorized list of data sources commonly used in program evaluation:

---

1. Student Performance Data

- **NCLEX-RN Pass Rates**: *National Council of State Boards of Nursing* (NCSBN) data detailing licensure examination success rates.
- **Graduation Rates**: Percentage of students completing the nursing program within the expected time frame.
- **Retention Rates**: Data on students persisting in the program across semesters or years.
- **Clinical Competency Evaluations**: Performance assessments during clinical rotations using standardized tools.
- **Course Grades and GPA**: Aggregated data reflecting academic performance across the program.

2. Faculty and Staff Data

- **Faculty Qualifications**: Documentation of degrees, certifications, and clinical expertise.
- **Faculty Workload Data**: Information on teaching hours, clinical supervision, and administrative duties.
- **Professional Development Records**: Evidence of continuing education, research involvement, and conference participation.
- **Faculty Evaluations**: Feedback from students, peers, and administrators on teaching effectiveness and mentorship.

3. Curriculum Data

- **Curriculum Maps**: Detailed documentation of how courses align with program goals and accreditation standards.

- **Syllabus Reviews**: Information on course objectives, content, and assessment methods.
- **Alignment with Accreditation Standards**: Data on how the curriculum meets national benchmarks (e.g., AACN Essentials).
- **Student Feedback**: Surveys and focus groups evaluating course content, teaching quality, and clinical training.

4. Clinical Education Data

- **Clinical Placement Records**: Details of partnerships with healthcare facilities, student placement, and rotation schedules.
- **Preceptor Feedback**: Evaluations from clinical preceptors regarding student preparedness and performance.
- **Simulation Lab Data**: Metrics on simulation usage, scenarios completed, and student outcomes during practice.

5. Employment and Post-Graduation Data

- **Employment Rates**: Percentage of graduates employed in nursing within six months of program completion.
- **Graduate Surveys**: Feedback on how well the program prepared alumni for professional roles.
- **Employer Feedback**: Insights from employers regarding graduate readiness, skill levels, and performance.

6. Student Support Services Data

- **Advising Records**: Data on academic advising sessions, student satisfaction, and outcomes.
- **Tutoring and Remediation Usage**: Metrics on participation in support services and their impact on student success.
- **Mental Health and Counseling Data**: Aggregated data on student use of counseling services and perceived support.

7. Stakeholder Feedback

- **Student Surveys and Focus Groups**: Regular evaluations are conducted by current students regarding their experience in the program.
- **Alumni Feedback**: Insights from graduates about the long-term value and impact of their education.
- **Community Partners**: Input from healthcare organizations on collaboration and alignment with workforce needs.

8. Program Outcomes Data

- **Accreditation Reports**: Feedback from accrediting agencies regarding compliance with standards and recommendations for improvement.
- **Program Improvement Plans**: Records of past actions to address deficiencies or enhance quality.
- **Outcome Trend Analysis**: Longitudinal data on key performance indicators, such as NCLEX pass rates and employment trends.

9. Institutional Data

- **Enrollment and Demographics**: Data on student diversity, including age, ethnicity, gender, and prior educational experience.
- **Institutional Resources**: Information on funding, facilities, and technological support.
- **Financial Aid Utilization**: Data on student use of scholarships, grants, and other funding sources.

10. Benchmarking and External Data

- **National Benchmarks**: Comparative data from sources like AACN, NCSBN, and regional accrediting bodies.
- **Peer Institution Comparisons**: Data comparing program outcomes with similar nursing programs.
- **Healthcare Trends**: Information on evolving industry demands and expectations for nursing graduates.

11. Program Evaluation Tools and Systems

- **Learning Management Systems (LMS)**: Data on course participation, grades, and assignment completion.
- **Student Information Systems (SIS)**: Comprehensive student records, including admissions, enrollment, and academic progress.
- **Clinical Management Software**: Data on clinical placement scheduling, evaluations, and hours logged.
- **Accreditation Management Platforms**: Tools for organizing and submitting data to accrediting bodies.

12. Continuous Improvement Data

- **Action Plan Progress Reports**: Documentation of steps taken to address identified areas for improvement.

- **Stakeholder Meetings**: Minutes and feedback from advisory boards, faculty meetings, and community partner collaborations.
- **Quality Improvement Metrics**: Data tracking progress on key improvement initiatives, such as retention efforts or curriculum updates.

Appendix B
Sample Evaluation Plan for Faculty and Student Participation in Program Governance in Nursing Programs

Introduction

Program governance in nursing education is vital for ensuring faculty and students contribute meaningfully to decision-making processes. This evaluation plan outlines how faculty and student participation in governance will be assessed to ensure inclusivity, effectiveness, and alignment with accreditation standards.

1. Objectives of the Evaluation Plan

- Assess the extent of faculty and student involvement in governance committees.
- Evaluate the effectiveness of communication between governance bodies and participants.
- Identify barriers to participation and recommend strategies to enhance engagement.
- Ensure compliance with accreditation standards that emphasize shared governance.

2. Key Stakeholders

- Faculty: Full-time and adjunct nursing faculty involved in program planning and policy-making.
- Students: Undergraduate and graduate nursing students participating in governance bodies or committees.
- Administrators: Program directors, department heads, and accreditation coordinators.

3. Evaluation Metrics

The following metrics will be used to measure participation and impact:

Faculty Metrics:

- **Participation Rates**: Percentage of faculty attending governance meetings.
- **Role Diversity**: Representation of full-time, adjunct, and tenured faculty in committees.
- **Contributions**: Number of agenda items proposed by faculty and adopted policies.
- **Satisfaction**: Survey results on faculty perceptions of their role in governance.

Student Metrics:

- **Participation Rates**: Percentage of student representatives attending meetings.
- **Diversity**: Representation of various cohorts, including undergraduates and graduates.
- **Engagement**: Frequency of student-led proposals or contributions to discussions.
- **Awareness**: Percentage of students who are aware of governance opportunities through surveys.

4. Data Collection Methods

Quantitative Methods:

1. **Attendance Records**: Track faculty and student attendance at governance meetings.
2. **Committee Reports**: Review meeting minutes for evidence of faculty and student contributions.
3. **Surveys**: Distribute surveys to faculty and students to measure participation satisfaction and perceived value.

Qualitative Methods:

1. **Focus Groups**: Conduct focus groups with faculty and students to gather insights on experiences and barriers.
2. **Interviews**: Interview committee chairs to evaluate the effectiveness of faculty and student input.

5. Data Analysis

- **Quantitative Analysis**: Use descriptive statistics (percentages, averages) to analyze attendance rates and survey results.
- **Qualitative Analysis**: Thematic analysis of focus group and interview transcripts to identify recurring themes related to participation barriers and successes.

6. Evaluation Timeline

Activity	Timeframe	Responsible Party
Develop evaluation tools	Month 1	Evaluation Committee
Distribute surveys	Month 2	Administrative assistant
Conduct focus groups	Months 2-3	External evaluator
Analyze data	Month 4	Data analysis team
Present findings and action plan	Month 5	Governance Committee

7. Reporting and Dissemination

- **Internal Reports**: Share findings with faculty, student representatives, and administrators during governance meetings.
- **Public Summary**: Develop a summary report for dissemination through program newsletters or the institutional website.

8. Action Plan

Based on evaluation results, the following actions will be taken:

- **Faculty Development**: Offer training on shared governance roles and responsibilities.
- **Student Engagement**: Create peer mentorship programs to guide students in governance roles.
- **Communication Improvements**: Regularly update all participants on governance activities and outcomes.
- **Policy Revisions**: Adjust governance structures to enhance inclusivity and participation.

9. Evaluation Success Indicators

- **Increased Participation**: A 20% increase in attendance rates among faculty and students within one year.
- **Improved Satisfaction**: At least 80% of survey respondents express satisfaction with their governance roles.

- **Enhanced Policy Contributions**: A measurable increase in policies and initiatives proposed by faculty and students.

Appendix C
Sample Evaluation Plan for Faculty Experience and Expertise in Program Governance in Nursing Programs

Introduction

Faculty expertise and experience are essential for effective program governance in nursing education. This evaluation plan provides a structured approach to assessing faculty members' qualifications, roles, and contributions to governance to ensure compliance with accreditation standards and the program's mission.

1. Objectives of the Evaluation Plan

- Evaluate the qualifications and governance experience of nursing faculty.
- Assess the effectiveness of faculty contributions to governance processes and decision-making.
- Identify areas where faculty development is needed to enhance governance expertise.
- Ensure alignment with accreditation standards related to faculty roles and governance.

2. Key Stakeholders

- **Faculty Members**: Full-time, part-time, and adjunct nursing faculty involved in governance.
- **Program Leadership**: Program directors, department chairs, and governance committee chairs.
- **Accreditation Committees**: Institutional accreditation coordinators and program evaluation teams.

3. Evaluation Metrics

The following metrics will be used to measure faculty expertise and experience:

Faculty Qualifications:

- **Educational Background**: Percentage of faculty with terminal degrees (e.g., PhD, DNP).

180

- **Certifications**: Number of faculty holding certifications relevant to their governance roles.
- **Years of Experience**: Average years of teaching and governance experience.
- **Boards of Nursing**: Number and percentage of faculty with requisite education and experience to qualify as a program director/instructor/assistant instructor.

Faculty Contributions:

- **Governance Roles**: Number of faculty serving as chairs or co-chairs in committees.
- **Policy Input**: Frequency of faculty-proposed initiatives adopted into policy.
- **Engagement**: Attendance rates and active participation in governance meetings.

Faculty Development:

- **Professional Development**: Participation in training sessions related to governance.
- **Satisfaction with Governance Roles**: Survey results measuring faculty satisfaction with their governance responsibilities.
- **Perceived Preparedness**: Faculty self-assessments on their readiness for governance roles.

4. Data Collection Methods

Quantitative Methods:

1. **Faculty Records**: Review CVs to assess qualifications, certifications, and governance experience.
2. **Attendance Logs**: Track participation rates in governance meetings and subcommittees.
3. **Surveys**: Distribute structured surveys to evaluate faculty satisfaction and perceived contributions.
4. **Boards of Nursing Records**: Review the status of faculty that fills roles as required by regulatory requirements.

Qualitative Methods:

1. **Interviews**: Conduct interviews with faculty members to explore their governance experiences and challenges.

2. **Meeting Minutes**: Analyze records of governance meetings to document faculty input and outcomes.
3. **Focus Groups**: Facilitate discussions to gather in-depth feedback on faculty roles in governance.

5. Data Analysis

- **Quantitative Analysis**: Use descriptive statistics to calculate percentages, averages, and participation rates.
- **Qualitative Analysis**: Thematic analysis of interview and focus group transcripts to identify strengths, barriers, and opportunities for improvement.

6. Evaluation Timeline

Activity	Timeframe	Responsible Party
Develop evaluation tools	Month 1	Program evaluation team
Distribute surveys	Month 2	Administrative Coordinator
Collect faculty records	Months 2-3	Human resources department
Conduct interviews and focus groups.	Months 3-4	External evaluator
Analyze data	Month 5	Data analysis team
Present findings	Month 6	Governance Committee

7. Reporting and Dissemination

- **Internal Reports**: Share findings with program leadership and governance committees during faculty retreats or department meetings.
- **Accreditation Reports**: Include evaluation outcomes in accreditation self-study documents.
- **Actionable Feedback**: Provide individual faculty members with personalized feedback and development plans.

8. Action Plan

Based on evaluation findings, the following actions will be implemented:

- **Faculty Development Programs**: Offer workshops on governance roles, decision-making, and leadership.

- **Mentorship Initiatives**: Pair less experienced faculty with seasoned governance leaders for skill-building.
- **Policy Adjustments**: Update governance policies to clarify faculty roles and expectations.

9. Evaluation Success Indicators

- **Improved Expertise**: Increase the percentage of faculty with certifications or additional training in governance-related skills.
- **Higher Engagement**: A 15% improvement in attendance and participation rates within one year.
- **Satisfaction Growth**: At least 80% of surveyed faculty reports improved satisfaction with governance roles.
- **Policy Contributions**: Increase in faculty-led initiatives successfully implemented in program governance.

Appendix D
Sample Evaluation Plan for Curriculum Assessment in Nursing Programs

Introduction

Curriculum assessment ensures nursing programs meet educational standards, produce competent graduates, and align with accreditation requirements. This evaluation plan outlines the steps and methodologies for systematically and effectively assessing the nursing curriculum.

---

1. Objectives of the Evaluation Plan

- Assess the alignment of the nursing curriculum with accreditation standards and professional competencies.
- Evaluate the effectiveness of the curriculum in achieving student learning outcomes (SLOs).
- Identify areas for curriculum improvement based on stakeholder feedback and outcome data.
- Ensure the curriculum reflects current trends and evidence-based practices in nursing education.

2. Key Stakeholders

- **Faculty**: Curriculum designers, course coordinators, and instructors.
- **Students**: Current nursing students and recent graduates.
- **Program Leadership**: Deans, directors, and accreditation liaisons.
- **External Stakeholders**: Employers, clinical site supervisors, and alumni.

3. Evaluation Metrics

The following metrics will measure the quality and effectiveness of the curriculum:

Curriculum Content:

- **Relevance**: Percentage of courses aligned with national benchmarks, such as the *AACN Essentials* and NCLEX-RN test plan.

- **Coverage of Competencies**: The extent to which the curriculum addresses core competencies, including patient care, communication, leadership, and evidence-based practice.

Student Outcomes:

- **NCLEX-RN Pass Rates**: Percentage of graduates passing the licensure exam on the first attempt.
- **Clinical Competency**: Student performance evaluations from clinical placements.

Stakeholder Feedback:

- **Student Satisfaction**: Survey results on the relevance and clarity of course content.
- **Employer Feedback**: Ratings on graduate preparedness for clinical practice.
- **Alumni Feedback**: Alumni self-assessments of the curriculum's effectiveness in their career readiness.

Program Responsiveness:

- **Curriculum Updates**: Frequency and scope of updates to reflect advances in nursing education and healthcare.
- **Integration of Technology**: Use of simulation, telehealth, and other innovative tools in teaching.

4. Data Collection Methods

Quantitative Methods:

1. **Student Performance Data**: Analyze course grades, NCLEX-RN pass rates, and clinical evaluation scores.
2. **Survey Instruments**: Use Likert-scale surveys to gather feedback from students, alumni, and employers.

Qualitative Methods:

1. **Focus Groups**: Discuss with students and faculty to explore perceptions of curriculum strengths and weaknesses.
2. **Content Analysis**: Review syllabi and instructional materials to assess alignment with accreditation standards.

5. Evaluation Activities and Timeline

Activity	Timeframe	Responsible Party
Curriculum mapping	Months 1-2	Curriculum Committee
Stakeholder surveys	Month 3	Program evaluation team
Focus groups with students	Month 4	External evaluator
Analysis of NCLEX-RN outcomes	Month 4	Data analyst
Syllabus review	Month 5	Faculty Subcommittee
Report preparation	Month 6	Program leadership

6. Data Analysis

- **Quantitative Analysis**: Use statistical software to analyze student performance metrics, survey responses, and NCLEX-RN pass rates.
- **Qualitative Analysis**: Employ thematic analysis for focus group transcripts and content reviews to identify patterns in stakeholder feedback.

7. Reporting and Dissemination

- **Internal Reports**: Share findings with faculty and program leadership during faculty meetings and retreats.
- **External Reporting**: Include evaluation outcomes in accreditation self-study reports.
- **Actionable Insights**: Provide specific recommendations for curriculum revisions based on data trends.

8. Action Plan for Improvement

- **Course Redesign**: Update or restructure courses with identified content or learning outcomes gaps.
- **Professional Development**: Train faculty in innovative teaching methods like active learning and technology integration.
- **Student Support Services**: Enhance tutoring and mentorship programs to address areas of student difficulty.

9. Success Indicators

- **Improved Outcomes**: Increase NCLEX-RN pass rates by at least 5% within two years.

- **Stakeholder Satisfaction**: Achieve at least 85% positive feedback from surveys on curriculum relevance and effectiveness.
- **Curriculum Alignment**: Ensure 100% of courses align with national benchmarks and professional standards.

Appendix E
Sample Evaluation Plan for Assessment of Physical Resources and Facilities in Nursing Programs

Introduction

The quality and availability of physical resources and facilities are critical to the success of nursing programs. This evaluation plan provides a structured approach to assess whether resources such as simulation labs, classrooms, clinical equipment, and technology meet the program's educational objectives and accreditation requirements.

1. Objectives of the Evaluation Plan

- Evaluate the adequacy and accessibility of physical resources to support learning outcomes and program growth.
- Assess the alignment of facilities with accreditation standards, such as those set by the ACEN and AACN.
- Identify gaps in resources and recommend improvements to enhance educational quality.
- Ensure compliance with health and safety regulations for physical spaces.

2. Key Stakeholders

- **Faculty**: Responsible for utilizing resources in teaching and learning.
- **Students**: Primary users of facilities and equipment.
- **Program Leadership**: Administrators managing resource allocation and budget.
- **Accrediting Bodies**: Require documentation of adequate resources and facilities.

3. Evaluation Metrics

Resource Adequacy:

- **Classroom Capacity**: Number of available classrooms and their seating capacity relative to enrollment numbers.

- **Simulation Labs**: Number of functional manikins, fidelity of simulations (high, medium, low), and hours of lab availability.
- **Clinical Equipment**: Quantity and condition of essential tools like IV pumps, monitors, and personal protective equipment.

Technology and Accessibility:

- **Technology Integration**: Availability of computers, projectors, and virtual learning platforms.
- **Wi-Fi Connectivity**: Coverage and reliability in all instructional areas.
- **Accessibility Compliance**: ADA-compliant entrances, elevators, and restroom facilities.

Satisfaction and Effectiveness:

- **Student Satisfaction**: Feedback on facilities' adequacy and usability.
- **Faculty Feedback**: Input on the impact of resources on teaching effectiveness.
- **Outcome Correlation**: Relationship between resource quality and student performance metrics, such as NCLEX-RN pass rates.

4. Data Collection Methods

Quantitative Methods:

1. **Resource Inventory**: Document all physical resources' number, type, and condition.
2. **Utilization Rates**: Track the frequency of lab, classroom, and equipment usage.

Qualitative Methods:

1. **Surveys**: Gather perceptions from students and faculty on the sufficiency and quality of resources.
2. **Focus Groups**: Conduct in-depth discussions with stakeholders to identify specific challenges or needs.
3. **Site Inspections**: Perform walk-through evaluations to assess resource availability, functionality, and safety.

5. Evaluation Activities and Timeline

Activity	Timeframe	Responsible Party
Conduct resource inventory	Month 1	Facilities Coordinator
Survey students and faculty	Month 2	Program evaluation team
Perform site inspections	Month 3	External evaluator
Analyze utilization rates	Month 3	Data analyst
Compile findings and recommendations.	Month 4	Program leadership

6. Data Analysis

- **Quantitative Analysis**: Use descriptive statistics to analyze resource availability, utilization rates, and survey responses.
- **Qualitative Analysis**: Apply thematic analysis to focus groups and survey comments to identify recurring issues or gaps.

7. Reporting and Dissemination

- **Internal Reports**: Present findings to faculty and program leadership during quarterly meetings.
- **Accreditation Documentation**: Include resource assessment data in self-study reports for accreditation reviews.
- **Public Reporting**: Share highlights with students and stakeholders to promote transparency.

8. Action Plan for Improvement

- **Resource Upgrades**: Allocate funds for replacing outdated equipment and expanding facilities.
- **Facility Enhancements**: Renovate classrooms and labs to improve accessibility and safety.
- **Technology Investments**: Incorporate advanced simulation technologies and ensure Wi-Fi coverage in all learning areas.
- **Policy Updates**: Establish policies for regular maintenance and facilities updates.

9. Success Indicators

- **Improved Satisfaction**: Achieve at least 90% positive feedback from students and faculty regarding facilities.

- **Enhanced Resource Utilization**: Ensure all simulation labs and clinical equipment are fully operational and accessible during scheduled hours.
- **Accreditation Compliance**: Meet or exceed accreditation standards for physical resources and facilities.

Appendix F
Sample Evaluation Plan for the Assessment of Adequate Faculty and Support Staffing in Nursing Programs

Introduction

Adequate faculty and support staffing are essential to ensure the delivery of high-quality nursing education. Faculty must meet qualification and workload standards, while support staff must provide administrative, clinical coordination, and technological assistance. This evaluation plan outlines a structured approach to assessing staffing adequacy, identifying gaps, and implementing improvements to align with accreditation standards and program objectives.

---

1. Objectives of the Evaluation Plan

- Evaluate the adequacy of faculty and support staff in meeting student and program needs.
- Assess faculty qualifications, workload, and availability against accreditation standards.
- Measure the sufficiency and effectiveness of support staff in administrative and clinical roles.
- Identify areas requiring adjustments to staffing levels or distribution.

2. Key Evaluation Questions

1. Does the program have sufficient faculty to maintain recommended student-to-faculty ratios in classroom and clinical settings?
2. Are faculty qualifications aligned with the program's academic and clinical goals?
3. Does the workload distribution allow faculty to balance teaching, research, and administrative duties effectively?
4. Is there adequate support staff to handle administrative, clinical, and technological needs?
5. How does the current staffing impact student outcomes, such as retention and NCLEX pass rates?

3. Metrics and Indicators

Faculty Metrics:

- **Student-to-Faculty Ratios**: Evaluate against national benchmarks, such as 1:8 for clinical settings.
- **Qualifications**: Percentage of faculty with advanced degrees (MSN, DNP, PhD) or certifications.
- **Workload Distribution**: Average teaching hours, clinical supervision, and administrative responsibilities per semester.
- **Faculty Retention**: Annual turnover rate and reasons for faculty departures.

Support Staff Metrics:

- **Administrative Support**: Ratio of students to administrative staff members.
- **Clinical Coordination**: Availability of staff to secure and manage clinical placements.
- **Technological Support**: Number of staff supporting simulation labs and learning management systems.

4. Data Collection Methods

Quantitative Data:

1. **Faculty and Staff Ratios**: Calculate the number of students per faculty and support staff.
2. **Qualifications Inventory**: Review faculty credentials and certifications.
3. **Retention and Turnover Rates**: Gather historical data on faculty and staff retention.
4. **Student Performance Metrics**: Analyze NCLEX pass, retention, and graduation rates.

Qualitative Data:

1. **Surveys**: Administer surveys to faculty, staff, and students about perceptions of staffing adequacy.
2. **Focus Groups**: Discuss with faculty and staff to understand workload and resource challenges.
3. **Exit Interviews**: Collect feedback from departing faculty and staff about staffing-related issues.

5. Timeline for Evaluation

Activity	Timeframe	Responsible Party
Data collection and analysis	Months 1–2	Program evaluation team
Faculty and staff surveys	Month 2	HR and program leadership
Focus groups and interviews	Month 3	External evaluator
Report drafting and review	Month 4	Accreditation Coordinator

6. Data Analysis

- **Quantitative Analysis**: Compare staffing levels, qualifications, and ratios to accreditation standards and national averages. Use statistical methods to identify significant gaps or trends.
- **Qualitative Analysis**: Identify recurring themes from survey and focus group feedback, focusing on workload challenges, resource availability, and staff satisfaction.

7. Reporting and Dissemination

- **Internal Report**: Share findings with program leadership, faculty, and administrative staff.
- **Stakeholder Presentation**: Summarize results for students, accrediting bodies, and external partners.
- **Accreditation Documentation**: Include findings in self-study reports or periodic accreditation updates.

8. Action Plan for Improvement

1. **Increase Staffing Levels**: Hire additional faculty and support staff to meet program growth or accreditation requirements.
2. **Faculty Development**: Provide funding for professional development and advanced certifications.
3. **Redistribute Workload**: Adjust teaching assignments or hire adjunct faculty to alleviate faculty workloads.
4. **Enhance Support Staff Resources**: Invest in technology and administrative training to optimize support staff roles.

9. Success Indicators

- **Compliance**: Achieve student-to-faculty and student-to-support staff ratios that meet or exceed accreditation standards.

- **Faculty Satisfaction**: Report 85% satisfaction with workload and support in faculty surveys.
- **Retention Rates**: Maintain a faculty and staff retention rate of 90% or higher annually.
- **Student Outcomes**: Demonstrate improvements in NCLEX pass rates and student satisfaction scores.

Appendix G
Checklist for Site Visit Preparation

Introduction

Preparing for an accreditation site visit is a crucial step in maintaining and renewing the accreditation of a nursing program. A successful site visit is grounded in meticulous planning, clear communication, and thorough documentation. Below is a comprehensive checklist that incorporates key steps for preparing your nursing program for a site visit, derived from the information in the chapters:

1. Pre-Visit Preparation

Alignment with Accreditation Standards

- ☐ Review the latest accreditation standards for your nursing program (e.g., ACEN, CCNE).
- ☐ Confirm that your program's mission, goals, and student learning outcomes align with the accreditation body's expectations.
- ☐ Ensure that your curriculum meets national benchmarks, such as those from AACN, and addresses areas like interprofessional collaboration and emerging healthcare trends (e.g., telehealth).
- ☐ Verify that faculty qualifications are up-to-date, including advanced degrees and ongoing professional development.

Gather Required Documentation

- ☐ **Program Mission, Goals, and Objectives**: Ensure the mission is well-documented and aligned with accreditation standards and national healthcare priorities.
- ☐ **Curriculum Maps and Syllabi**: Ensure syllabi reflect program goals, student outcomes, and course objectives.
- ☐ **Faculty Credentials**: Collect and organize CVs, certifications, and evidence of ongoing professional development.
- ☐ **Student and Faculty Evaluations**: Compile data on program evaluations, faculty performance reviews, and student surveys.
- ☐ **Program Outcomes**: Gather data on NCLEX-RN pass rates, graduation rates, employment outcomes, and retention rates.

- ☐ **Student Support Services**: Provide documentation detailing advising, counseling, clinical placements, and mentorship programs.
- ☐ **Program Evaluation and Continuous Improvement**: Organize records of program evaluations, improvement plans, and annual reviews.

Assign Key Personnel to Prepare for Interviews

- ☐ Assign program directors, faculty, and staff to prepare for interviews with the site visit team.
- ☐ Ensure faculty and administrators are well-versed in accreditation standards, program goals, and recent improvements.
- ☐ Identify student representatives or alumni who can discuss the program's strengths and outcomes.

2. Preparing the Campus and Facilities

Ensure Campus Readiness

- ☐ Review campus facilities, including classrooms, clinical labs, simulation areas, and student study spaces.
- ☐ Ensure clinical placement sites (e.g., hospitals, clinics) are properly documented and aligned with accreditation standards.
- ☐ Conduct a walkthrough of the campus and facilities to ensure cleanliness, accessibility, and functionality for site visitors.

Organize Campus Tour Logistics

- ☐ Develop a campus tour itinerary highlighting key spaces relevant to the accreditation visit (e.g., simulation labs, classrooms, student support areas).
- ☐ Designate knowledgeable staff or faculty to serve as tour guides and provide insights into how spaces contribute to student learning and program objectives.

3. Coordinating Logistics for Site Visit

Establish a Site Visit Schedule

- ☐ Develop a detailed schedule that outlines the site visit dates, times for interviews, campus tours, and review of documents.
- ☐ Include times for individual and group meetings with stakeholders such as faculty, students, administrators, and clinical partners.

    ☐   Ensure that all site visitors are included in the schedule and that there is sufficient time for questions and discussions.

Prepare a Welcome Package for the Site Visit Team

    ☐   Prepare a welcome package that includes:
- A detailed schedule of the visit.
- Information about your program and the campus (e.g., program history, student demographics, community partnerships).
- Copies of key documents (e.g., mission statement, accreditation reports, outcome data).
- A map of the campus and facilities.

4. Preparing Key Stakeholders for Interviews and Discussions

Prepare Faculty for Interviews

    ☐   Discuss with faculty the goals of the site visit and what accreditation representatives will be evaluating (e.g., teaching effectiveness, faculty qualifications, curriculum design).

    ☐   Provide faculty with a brief on effectively communicating the program's strengths, successes, and areas for improvement.

Prepare Students for Interviews

    ☐   Ensure that students understand the role they play in the accreditation process.

    ☐   Provide students with an overview of the program's mission and outcomes, encouraging them to share their experiences with faculty and the program overall.

Prepare Administrators and Stakeholders

    ☐   Prepare program administrators and key staff to articulate how the program meets accreditation standards, particularly in financial resources, faculty development, and continuous improvement efforts.

5. Review the Site Visit Guidelines

Familiarize with Accreditation Expectations

☐ Review the site visit guidelines and expectations the accrediting body provides (e.g., ACEN, CCNE).

☐ Understand the expectations for documentation, interviews, and site visit protocol.

Anticipate Potential Questions

☐ Prepare for questions about the following areas:
  - Program outcomes (e.g., NCLEX pass, employment, graduation rates).
  - Curriculum design and assessment methods.
  - Student support services (e.g., advising, clinical placements, tutoring).
  - Faculty qualifications, professional development, and teaching strategies.
  - Program evaluation and continuous improvement processes.

Prepare for Challenges or Areas of Improvement

☐ Be ready to discuss areas where the program may have challenges or is in the process of improvement.

☐ Have documentation and action plans in place to demonstrate how these challenges are being addressed (e.g., student retention issues and curriculum updates).

6. Communication and Documentation During the Visit

Prepare for Site Visit Communication

☐ Ensure that all stakeholders (faculty, staff, students) are informed about the visit and their roles in the process.

☐ Communicate clearly to all involved that the purpose of the site visit is to provide constructive feedback and ensure continuous improvement.

Document All Interactions

☐ Keep detailed records of the site visit, including meeting notes, feedback from the site visit team, and any additional requests for information or clarification.

7. Post-Visit Actions

Debrief and Evaluate the Visit

- ☐ After the site visit, faculty and administrators will be debriefed to discuss the feedback received.
- ☐ Review the recommendations from the site visit and develop a plan to address them.

Prepare for Final Report Submission

- ☐ Ensure all required documents and evidence are submitted to the accrediting agency, including the site visit team's feedback, recommendations, and corrective action plans.
- ☐ Address all areas of non-compliance or improvement and provide a clear timeline for resolving issues.

Appendix H
Sample Communication Plan for Stakeholders

Stakeholder Communication Plan for Accreditation Site Visit

Purpose

To ensure all stakeholders are well-informed, engaged, and prepared for the accreditation site visit, fostering transparency, collaboration, and compliance with accreditation standards.

Stakeholder Groups

1. **Internal Stakeholders**:

   o   Faculty and Staff

   o   Students

   o   Administrative Leadership

   o   Support Staff

2. **External Stakeholders**:

   o   Clinical Partners

   o   Alumni

   o   Employers

   o   Accrediting Body Representatives

Communication Objectives

- Ensure clarity about accreditation standards and site visit expectations.
- Provide a platform for stakeholder input and collaboration.
- Maintain transparency and trust throughout the process.

- Align stakeholder actions and responses with accreditation goals.

Communication Methods

- **Meetings and Workshops**:

    - Faculty/staff preparation workshops (curriculum alignment, evidence review).

    - Student and alumni town halls to address their roles and expectations.

- **Emails and Newsletters**:

    - Regular updates on site visit schedules, milestones, and required documentation.

    - FAQs about the accreditation process for stakeholders.

- **Web Portals**:

    - A dedicated accreditation section on the nursing program's website for updates and resources.

- **One-on-One Consultations**:

    - Personalized sessions for faculty or clinical partners to address specific responsibilities.

- **Mock Interviews and Sessions**:

    - Simulated sessions to prepare stakeholders for site visit interactions.

Timeline and Milestones

Timeline	Activity
6 Months Before	Initial stakeholder briefing, form accreditation committees.
3 Months Before	Begin targeted training sessions for faculty, staff, and clinical partners.

Timeline	Activity
1 Month Before	Finalize documentation and conduct mock site visit evaluations.
1 Week Before	Share finalized agenda and reminders with all stakeholders.
Day of Visit	Provide real-time updates and ensure stakeholder availability.

Key Messages

1. Accreditation affirms program quality and aligns with industry standards.

2. Stakeholders play a vital role in demonstrating program strengths and addressing questions.

3. Open communication and collaboration will ensure a successful visit.

Evaluation and Follow-Up

- Distribute post-visit surveys to stakeholders for feedback on communication efficacy.

- Conduct a debrief session to summarize findings and discuss continuous improvement strategies.

This plan should adapt as specific stakeholder needs or accrediting body requirements are identified.

Appendix I
Sample Kick-off Meeting Agenda

Agenda: Initial Informational Kick-Off Meeting with Stakeholders

Purpose: To provide an overview of the accreditation site visit, explain roles and expectations, and initiate stakeholder engagement in the preparation process.

Meeting Details

- **Date:** [Insert Date]
- **Time:** [Insert Time]
- **Location:** [Insert Location or Virtual Meeting Link]
- **Facilitator:** [Name/Title, e.g., Accreditation Coordinator]

Agenda

1. Welcome and Introductions (10 minutes)

- **Facilitator:** [Insert Name]
  - ○ Welcome attendees.
  - ○ Brief introduction of accreditation team and stakeholders.
  - ○ Purpose of the meeting.

2. Overview of Accreditation and Its Importance (15 minutes)

- **Presenter:** [Insert Name, e.g., Dean of Nursing]
  - ○ Accreditation purpose and significance for the program, students, and institution.
  - ○ Key accrediting body (e.g., ACEN or CCNE) standards.
  - ○ Benefits of achieving accreditation.

3. Accreditation Process and Timeline (20 minutes)

- **Presenter:** [Insert Name, e.g., Accreditation Liaison]

  - Summary of the accreditation process, including self-study, site visit, and decision phases.

  - Key milestones and deadlines leading up to the site visit.

  - Highlight the importance of stakeholder engagement in the process.

4. Roles and Responsibilities of Stakeholders (20 minutes)

- **Presenter:** [Insert Name, e.g., Faculty Lead or Clinical Coordinator]

  - Expectations for faculty, staff, students, clinical partners, and alumni.

  - Overview of evidence/documentation needed from each group.

  - Role of stakeholders during the site visit (e.g., interviews, Q&A sessions).

5. Site Visit Preparation (15 minutes)

- **Presenter:** [Insert Name, e.g., Administrative Lead]

  - What to expect during the site visit.

  - Overview of mock site visit and readiness activities.

  - Guidelines for interacting with accreditors (e.g., professionalism, focus on program strengths).

6. Communication Plan and Resources (10 minutes)

- **Presenter:** [Insert Name, e.g., Communication Coordinator]

  - How stakeholders will receive updates (emails, newsletters, meetings).

  - Available resources: self-study documents, accreditation FAQs, and training sessions.

7. Q&A and Open Discussion (20 minutes)

- **Facilitator:** [Insert Name]

  - Open floor for stakeholder questions and concerns.

    o Gather initial feedback and suggestions.

8. Next Steps and Action Items (10 minutes)

- **Facilitator:** [Insert Name]

  - Review immediate action items and upcoming meetings.

  - Assign roles for data gathering, preparation tasks, and subcommittee participation.

  - Confirm follow-up timeline and contact points for questions.

9. Closing Remarks (5 minutes)

- **Facilitator:** [Insert Name]

  - Recap the importance of collaboration and shared goals.

  - Thank attendees for their commitment to the accreditation process.

Meeting Materials

- Handout: Accreditation process overview and timeline.

- FAQ document about accreditation and stakeholder roles.

- Contact information for accreditation team leads.

Expected Outcomes

- Stakeholders understand the accreditation process, their roles, and the preparation timeline.

- Questions and concerns are addressed to build confidence and engagement.

- Initial steps and action items are assigned to key stakeholders.

Appendix J
Sample Logistics and Coordination Plan

Purpose

To ensure seamless execution of the accreditation site visit, effectively coordinate all logistical elements, facilitate stakeholder communication, and ensure compliance with accrediting body requirements.

Plan Components

1. Site Visit Overview

- **Dates of Visit:** [Insert Dates]

- **Accreditation Team:** [Number of reviewers, names (if known)]

- **Primary Contact:** [Name, Title, Contact Information]

- **Visit Objectives:**

    o   Review of facilities, curriculum, and resources.

    o   Meetings with stakeholders (faculty, students, administrators, clinical partners).

    o   Verification of self-study documentation and compliance with accreditation standards.

2. Leadership Team

Role	Name	Responsibilities
Accreditation Coordinator	[Insert Name]	Primary point of contact; oversees logistics.
Facility Manager	[Insert Name]	Prepares physical spaces, technology, and signage.

Role	Name	Responsibilities
Communication Lead	[Insert Name]	Updates stakeholders and coordinates schedules.
Support Staff Lead	[Insert Name]	Assigns support roles for tasks like escorting reviewers or assisting during sessions.

3. Schedule and Agenda Coordination

- **Draft Agenda Development:**

  o Outline based on accrediting body requirements.

  o Include meetings with faculty, students, administration, and clinical partners.

- **Finalized Schedule:**

  o Circulate agenda to reviewers and stakeholders 2 weeks prior to the visit.

  o Assign responsible individuals to manage each segment of the schedule.

- **Time Allocation:**

  o Allow 15–30 minutes between sessions for transitions and flexibility.

4. Facility and Space Preparation

- **Primary Locations:**

  o Meeting rooms (administrative interviews, faculty meetings).

  o Classrooms or simulation labs (observations).

  o Conference rooms for document review.

- **Technology Needs:**

  o Ensure internet access, projectors, laptops, and video conferencing equipment are functional.

- o   Arrange for IT support on standby.

- **Signage:**

  - o   Clear directional signs for all meeting locations.

  - o   "Accreditation in Progress" signs to minimize disruptions.

---

5. Stakeholder Coordination

- **Faculty and Staff:**

  - o   Provide briefing sessions on expectations and potential questions.

  - o   Ensure availability for scheduled interviews and Q&A sessions.

- **Students:**

  - o   Select and prepare a representative group for discussions.

  - o   Share FAQs and sample questions to set expectations.

- **Clinical Partners and Alumni:**

  - o   Confirm participation and coordinate transportation (if needed).

  - o   Brief participants on their roles and topics of discussion.

---

6. Documentation and Evidence Management

- **Document Review Room:**

  - o   Reserve a dedicated space for accreditation reviewers to access materials.

  - o   Ensure copies of the self-study report, course syllabi, policy documents, and performance data are available (physical or electronic).

- **Compliance Checklists:**

  - o   Verify all requested documentation is accurate and accessible.

  - o   Assign a team member to be on-call for additional document requests during the visit.

7. Hospitality and Logistics

- **Transportation:**
  - o Arrange pick-up/drop-off services for reviewers if needed.
  - o Provide a map and directions to campus and key facilities.

- **Accommodation:**
  - o Reserve lodging for reviewers in proximity to the campus.
  - o Confirm reservations and provide reviewers with hotel details.

- **Meals and Refreshments:**
  - o Schedule catered meals (e.g., breakfast, lunch, coffee breaks).
  - o Provide a list of local dining options for reviewers during off-hours.

8. On-Site Coordination During Visit

Day of Visit	Task	Assigned Team Member
Welcome and Orientation	Greet reviewers, distribute welcome packets.	[Insert Name]
Session Management	Monitor meeting start/end times.	[Insert Name]
Escort Duties	Guide reviewers to/from locations.	[Insert Name]
IT/AV Support	Address any technical issues promptly.	[Insert Name]
Hospitality Point of Contact	Oversee catering and refreshments.	[Insert Name]

9. Contingency Planning

- **Technical Issues:**

  o Backup devices (e.g., laptops, projectors).

  o IT team on-call for immediate troubleshooting.

- **Schedule Changes:**

  o Flexible buffer slots in the schedule.

  o Contact list for immediate rescheduling communication.

- **Reviewer Needs:**

  o Provide an on-site liaison for special requests or last-minute changes.

10. Post-Visit Actions

- **Debrief Meeting:**

  o Conduct an internal meeting to review preliminary feedback and observations.

- **Thank You Notes:**

  o Send personalized thank-you emails or letters to reviewers and participating stakeholders.

- **Feedback Collection:**

  o Gather stakeholder input on the process for future improvement.

- **Follow-Up Reports:**

  o Address any concerns or requests for additional documentation promptly.

Key Contacts

Role	Name	Email	Phone
Accreditation Coordinator	[Insert Name]	[Insert Email]	[Insert Phone]

Role	Name	Email	Phone
IT Support Lead	[Insert Name]	[Insert Email]	[Insert Phone]
Logistics Coordinator	[Insert Name]	[Insert Email]	[Insert Phone]

This logistics and coordination plan ensures the accreditation site visit is well-organized, professional, and efficient, showcasing the nursing program's commitment to quality and compliance.

Appendix K
Key Resources for Nursing Program Accreditation

Successfully navigating the nursing program accreditation process requires access to a wide range of resources that guide programs through the necessary steps to achieve and maintain accreditation. Below is a list of key resources that nursing programs can utilize:

Accrediting Bodies and Agencies

- o **Accreditation Commission for Education in Nursing (ACEN)**
  Website: https://www.acenursing.org
  ACEN accredits nursing programs at all levels, ensuring they meet national standards for quality education.
- o **Commission on Collegiate Nursing Education (CCNE)**
  Website: https://www.aacnnursing.org/CCNE
  CCNE is a recognized accrediting agency that focuses on the quality and integrity of baccalaureate, graduate, and residency programs in nursing.
- o **National League for Nursing Commission for Nursing Education Accreditation (NLN CNEA)**
  Website: https://www.nln.org/cnea
  NLN CNEA accredits nursing programs in diploma, associate, baccalaureate, and graduate-level nursing programs, offering accreditation standards and process resources.

Professional Associations and Advocacy Groups

- o **American Association of Colleges of Nursing (AACN)**
  Website: https://www.aacnnursing.org
  AACN represents academic nursing and provides resources for nursing schools, including accreditation information, policy updates, and educational standards.
- o **National Council of State Boards of Nursing (NCSBN)**
  Website: https://www.ncsbn.org
  NCSBN offers resources and tools for nursing education, including NCLEX exam preparation, licensure requirements, and statistics on nursing education outcomes.

    o **American Nurses Association (ANA)**
Website: https://www.nursingworld.org
ANA supports nurses through advocacy, education, and
resources related to the practice of nursing and nursing
education.

Guides and Manuals for Accreditation

    o **ACEN Accreditation Manual**
Provides detailed information on ACEN accreditation
standards, processes, and procedures, helping programs prepare
for accreditation visits and submissions.
    o **CCNE Accreditation Handbook**
Offers guidance on the CCNE accreditation process, including
self-study preparation, evidence submission, and requirements
for sustaining accreditation.
    o **NLN CNEA Accreditation Standards**
A guide detailing the NLN's accreditation standards and criteria,
helping programs understand how to align their curriculum,
faculty, and student outcomes with national expectations.

Data and Analytics Tools

    o **National Center for Education Statistics (NCES)**
Website: https://nces.ed.gov
NCES provides key data on nursing education trends,
graduation rates, employment outcomes, and demographics,
helping programs benchmark their success.
    o **Integrated Postsecondary Education Data System (IPEDS)**
Website: https://nces.ed.gov/ipeds
IPEDS offers data related to U.S. higher education institutions,
including enrollment figures, graduation rates, and other key
performance indicators relevant to accreditation.

Accreditation Self-Study Templates and Tools

    o **ACEN Self-Study Guide**
ACEN provides a self-study guide to help programs document
compliance with accreditation standards, facilitating the self-
evaluation process before the site visit.
    o **CCNE Self-Study Templates**
Available to help nursing programs conduct thorough self-

assessments and prepare evidence for accreditation reviews, including assessing the alignment of program outcomes with national standards.

Clinical Placement Resources

- ○ **Nurse Practitioners in the Workplace (NPW) Network**
  Website: https://www.npw.org
  NPW is an online platform that connects nursing programs with clinical placement opportunities and facilitates the placement of students in high-quality clinical settings.
- ○ **Clinical Placement Network (CPN)**
  A resource that offers access to a database of clinical placement sites, helping programs locate quality practice sites for nursing students.

Quality Improvement and Program Development

- ○ **Institute for Healthcare Improvement (IHI)**
  Website: https://www.ihi.org
  IHI provides resources and tools for quality improvement, including strategies to enhance patient care and improve healthcare systems relevant to nursing programs seeking accreditation.
- ○ **Quality and Safety Education for Nurses (QSEN)**
  Website: https://qsen.org
  QSEN offers resources on integrating quality and safety competencies into nursing education, a key component of accreditation standards.

Faculty Development and Continuing Education

- ○ **American Association of Nurse Practitioners (AANP)**
  Website: https://www.aanp.org
  AANP provides continuing education opportunities, resources, and professional development for nursing faculty to maintain expertise and meet accreditation standards.
- ○ **National League for Nursing (NLN) Faculty Development Resources**
  Website: https://www.nln.org
  NLN offers a wealth of resources for faculty development,

including workshops, seminars, and online courses that align with accreditation requirements.

Technology and Simulation Resources

- ○ **Society for Simulation in Healthcare (SSH)**
  Website: https://www.ssih.org
  SSH provides accreditation for simulation-based education programs, offering tools and resources to enhance the use of simulation in nursing education.

Additional Accreditation-Related Research and Publications

- ○ **Nursing Education Perspectives (NEP)**
  Website: https://www.nln.org/nursing-education-perspectives
  A journal published by the National League for Nursing that offers research articles, best practices, and policy updates related to nursing education and accreditation.
- ○ **Journal of Nursing Education**
  Website: https://www.healio.com/nursing/journals/jne
  Provides peer-reviewed articles on the latest research in nursing education, including accreditation-related studies and developments.

Grants and Funding Resources

Accreditation can be a resource-intensive process, requiring significant financial investment. Below are some funding resources that may assist nursing programs with the costs associated with accreditation, program development, and improvement initiatives:

- • **Health Resources and Services Administration (HRSA) Nursing Workforce Development Grants**
  Website: https://bhw.hrsa.gov/funding-opportunities
  HRSA provides funding to support nursing education, practice, and retention programs, helping nursing schools with accreditation costs and faculty development.
- • **Robert Wood Johnson Foundation (RWJF)**
  Website: https://www.rwjf.org
  RWJF offers numerous grants related to nursing education, workforce development, and healthcare initiatives that align with accreditation goals.

- **National Institute of Nursing Research (NINR)**
  Website: https://www.ninr.nih.gov
  NINR offers grants for nursing research, which can improve faculty qualifications and contribute to the program's overall accreditation quality, particularly in advanced practice programs.

Nursing Simulation and Technology Resources

Technology plays a significant role in nursing education, particularly in simulation. Accredited programs often integrate simulation to meet both educational and clinical training standards.

- **International Nursing Association for Clinical Simulation and Learning (INACSL)**
  Website: https://www.inacsl.org
  INACSL provides resources, standards, and best practices for simulation in nursing education, including a framework for accreditation of simulation programs in nursing schools.
- **American Society for Clinical Pathology (ASCP) Simulation Resources**
  Website: https://www.ascp.org
  ASCP offers educational resources on clinical simulation, which can be vital for nursing programs aiming to meet accreditation standards for practical skills.

Continuous Improvement and Accreditation Tools

For continuous improvement, some tools can help nursing programs monitor, analyze, and improve educational outcomes in preparation for reaccreditation:

- **Plan-Do-Study-Act (PDSA) Cycle**
  Resource: Institute for Healthcare Improvement (IHI) - PDSA Cycle Overview
  This widely used framework helps nursing programs implement and track quality improvement processes, a key component of maintaining accreditation.
- **Nursing Education Quality Improvement Collaborative (NEQIC)**
  Website: https://www.aacnnursing.org
  NEQIC offers resources to improve nursing education programs through data collection, analysis, and quality improvement processes that align with accreditation standards.

Legal and Regulatory Resources

Staying up-to-date with changes in laws, regulations, and accreditation requirements is essential for nursing programs to ensure ongoing compliance.

- **National Association of Regulatory Boards of Nursing (NCSBN)**
  Website: https://www.ncsbn.org
  NCSBN provides comprehensive resources on licensure, certification, and regulation, as well as guidelines for the accreditation of nursing education programs to meet state and national requirements.
- **U.S. Department of Education (USDOE) Accreditation Guidelines**
  Website: https://www.ed.gov/accreditation
  The USDOE provides guidelines and recognition of accrediting agencies, supporting nursing programs in understanding federal accreditation standards and maintaining compliance.

Faculty Development and Support

Ongoing professional development of faculty is essential for maintaining high standards in nursing education. Several resources focus on enhancing faculty qualifications and teaching effectiveness, ensuring that programs meet accreditation standards.

- **The National League for Nursing (NLN) Center for Faculty Development**
  Website: https://www.nln.org
  NLN offers numerous workshops, webinars, and educational materials focused on faculty development, which can help programs align with accreditation standards related to teaching excellence.
- **American Association of Colleges of Nursing (AACN) Faculty Development Resources**
  Website: https://www.aacnnursing.org
  AACN provides resources, including faculty certification programs, grants, leadership development initiatives, and support programs to meet the accreditation standard for faculty expertise.

Peer Networks and Collaborative Resources

Accreditation is a dynamic process that benefits from collaboration with peer institutions. Many professional networks provide programs with access to shared knowledge, best practices, and peer review.

- **Council for Accreditation of Nurse Anesthesia Educational Programs (COA)**
  Website: https://www.coa.us.com
  COA provides specific accreditation guidelines and resources for nurse anesthesia programs, helping programs meet accreditation standards for specialized nursing education.
- **National Organization of Nurse Practitioner Faculties (NONPF)**
  Website: https://www.nonpf.org
  NONPF provides a network of nursing educators and a host of resources on advanced practice nursing education, supporting programs in achieving and maintaining accreditation.
- **State Nursing Organizations**
  Many states have nursing education organizations that provide resources, updates, and networking opportunities for nursing programs to stay informed about state-specific accreditation requirements.

Clinical Placement and Partnerships

Accrediting bodies often require nursing programs to establish partnerships with clinical settings. Building and maintaining these partnerships is crucial for meeting accreditation requirements.

- **Clinical Placement Network (CPN)**
  Website: https://www.clinicalplacementnetwork.com
  CPN connects nursing programs with clinical placement sites, helping to ensure that students meet accreditation requirements for clinical hours and experience.
- **University Health Systems and Medical Institutions**
  Local hospitals and health systems often partner with nursing programs to provide clinical placements and practice settings. Establishing formal agreements with these institutions is essential for program accreditation.

Accreditation Review and Evaluation Software

Several software platforms assist nursing programs in tracking their accreditation status, managing data collection, and preparing for review.

- **Nuventive Improve**
  Website: https://www.nuventive.com
  This platform allows programs to align data collection, strategic planning, and outcomes assessment to meet accreditation standards. It

helps in managing continuous quality improvement and accreditation requirements.

- **Watermark Analytics**
  Website: https://www.watermarkinsights.com
  Watermark offers tools that enable institutions to collect and analyze data to support accreditation efforts, including tracking course effectiveness, student learning outcomes, and faculty performance.

Answers to End of Chapter Questions

Chapter 1

1. b) To ensure that the program meets established standards for quality and effectiveness
2. b) Commission on Collegiate Nursing Education (CCNE)
3. c) Regional accreditation evaluates the overall institution, while programmatic accreditation evaluates the nursing program specifically.
4. b) Eligibility for federal funding and grants
5. b) A comprehensive internal assessment of the program's compliance with accreditation standards
6. b) To ensure that the program remains relevant, effective, and aligned with evolving healthcare needs
7. c) Difficulty in meeting accreditation standards related to curriculum design and faculty qualifications
8. b) Every 3 to 5 years
9. b) They play a key role in ensuring the program aligns with standards and contributing to the self-study and improvement initiatives.
10. b) Inability to demonstrate compliance with accreditation standards, such as faculty qualifications or curriculum rigor

1. established, professional
2. Commission on Collegiate Nursing Education
3. Regional, programmatic
4. Federal
5. self-study
6. site
7. continuous
8. student
9. 3, 5
10. Probationary

Chapter 2

1. Identifying the appropriate accrediting body is the first critical step, as different bodies have specific standards and processes to be followed for the program to gain and maintain accreditation. Choosing the correct accrediting body aligns the program with the right expectations and criteria.
2. The accreditation process typically involves conducting a self-study, preparing for a site visit, and undergoing a review by the accrediting body. The self-study involves an internal assessment of the program's strengths, weaknesses, and alignment with accreditation standards. The site visit includes an on-site review by an evaluation team, which involves a comprehensive assessment of all documentation and program outcomes.

3. Forming an internal team ensures that all necessary perspectives are considered when assessing the program's readiness for accreditation. Key stakeholders such as faculty, administrators, clinical partners, and student representatives should be included to ensure the process reflects all aspects of the program, from curriculum to resources and clinical training.

4. Key factors include understanding the accreditation body's deadlines, ensuring adequate time for gathering the necessary documentation, addressing areas of weakness, preparing for the site visit, and ensuring faculty and staff are adequately involved and trained throughout the process.

5. A gap analysis helps identify areas where the program does not meet accreditation standards. It provides a clear roadmap for improvements, ensuring that the program addresses these areas before applying for accreditation. This process helps avoid unnecessary delays or complications during the accreditation review.

6. Common challenges include limited resources, inadequate faculty development, and difficulty aligning the curriculum with accreditation standards. These can be mitigated by early planning, dedicating time and resources to faculty training, seeking external expertise if necessary, and fostering a culture of continuous improvement.

7. Program outcomes, such as graduation rates, NCLEX pass rates, and employment rates, demonstrate the effectiveness of the nursing program in preparing students for professional practice. These metrics are a key part of the accreditation review process, as they provide evidence of the program's success and alignment with accreditation standards.

8. The self-study is a comprehensive internal assessment of the nursing program, detailing how it meets or plans to meet accreditation standards. It should include an evaluation of faculty qualifications, curriculum, student outcomes, resources, and clinical partnerships, along with a clear action plan for addressing any areas of deficiency.

9. Stakeholder engagement is critical because accreditation affects various parties, including faculty, students, administrators, and clinical partners. Effective engagement can be achieved through regular communication, involvement in planning meetings, and ensuring stakeholders' feedback is incorporated into the preparation and improvement strategies.

10. Nursing programs can ensure they meet accrediting bodies' expectations by thoroughly reviewing accreditation standards, conducting a gap analysis, and aligning their mission, goals, and curriculum with those standards. At the same time, they should focus on leveraging their unique characteristics—such as innovative teaching methods, clinical partnerships, and community involvement—to enhance their program's value and distinctiveness.

1. accrediting body
2. self-study, site visit, review
3. perspectives
4. deadlines
5. gap analysis
6. self
7. effectiveness
8. stakeholder
9. improvement

10. site

Chapter 3

Multiple Choice Questions

1. B) To evaluate the program's alignment with accreditation standards
2. D) Marketing budget
3. B) Vision statement
4. B) Ensuring that evidence is based on data and aligned with accreditation standards
5. A) It helps create a cohesive and inclusive process

True/False Questions

6. False
7. True
8. False
9. True
10. False

Short Answer Questions

11. Explain the role of program outcomes in the self-study process for accreditation.
12. What common challenges do nursing programs face during self-study, and how can they be addressed?
13. Why is it important to align a nursing program's curriculum with accreditation standards, and what methods can be used to ensure this alignment?
14. What types of evidence are typically collected to support a nursing program's self-study, and how is this evidence used in the accreditation process?
15. Describe the role of faculty, staff, and students in the self-study process and explain why their engagement is essential for success.

Fill-in-the-Blank Questions

16. Mission
17. Gap
18. Continuous Quality Improvement (CQI)
19. Supporting
20. Accurate

Essay Question

21. The self-study process is critical to nursing program accreditation as it comprehensively assesses the program's alignment with established standards. The self-study's key components include the program's mission and vision, faculty qualifications, curriculum review, student outcomes, and support services. Data collection and evidence are central to demonstrating the program's effectiveness and areas for improvement. Faculty and staff engagement must ensure the process is collaborative, reflective, and thorough. Their insights contribute to a more accurate evaluation and a stronger case for

accreditation. Involving faculty and staff in the self-study process strengthens the documentation. It fosters a culture of continuous improvement that benefits the program in the long term.

Chapter 4

Multiple Choice Questions:

1. B. To assess the program's compliance with accreditation standards
2. C. Providing funding to the program
3. Ensuring faculty are aware of accreditation standards and expectations
4. Scheduling interviews and meetings with key stakeholders

True or False:

1. **False** (The program itself is responsible for creating the self-study document.)
2. **True**
3. **False** (Facilities should be prepared and available for review during the site visit.)
4. **True**

Short Answer Questions:

1. **Answer:** The site visit is critical because it allows the accrediting team to observe the program's operations, facilities, and adherence to accreditation standards. It also provides an opportunity to interview faculty, staff, and students to ensure the program meets quality education and patient care benchmarks.
2. **Answer:** Programs can prepare faculty by reviewing the accreditation standards, conducting mock interviews, ensuring faculty understand the program's strengths and areas for improvement, and encouraging them to be candid and transparent during the interviews. Faculty should also know their role in student outcomes, curriculum effectiveness, and overall program goals.
3. **Answer:** One potential challenge is inadequate documentation or incomplete evidence to support the program's compliance with accreditation standards. This can be avoided by thoroughly organizing and cross-checking all necessary documentation in advance, ensuring it is readily available for review by the accreditation team.
4. **Answer:** Logistical coordination ensures that the site visit runs smoothly by scheduling interviews, organizing campus tours, arranging meeting spaces, and facilitating clear communication between the program and the accreditation team. Well-managed logistics help to create a professional, organized atmosphere that demonstrates the program's commitment to the accreditation process.

4. Essay Questions:

1. **Answer:** Transparency is crucial during the site visit because it fosters trust between the program and the accreditation team. Being open about the program's strengths, weaknesses, and challenges allows the site visit team to assess the program's alignment with accreditation standards accurately. Transparency demonstrates the program's commitment to continuous improvement and ethical practices, which can positively influence the evaluation outcome. On the other hand, a lack of transparency can lead to skepticism from the accreditation team and may result in a negative review.

2. **Answer:** Preparing the campus and stakeholders ensures that everyone involved understands the importance of the site visit and is ready to engage in productive discussions. Faculty should be familiar with accreditation standards and prepared to discuss their teaching methods and how they contribute to student success. Key stakeholders, such as staff and administrators, should be prepared to demonstrate how their roles support the program's mission and goals. Well-prepared faculty and staff can provide accurate, positive, and evidence-based information during the interviews, which helps the site visit team evaluate thoroughly and favorably. Additionally, having a well-organized campus and accessible documentation creates a professional and efficient experience, which reflects positively on the program's readiness for accreditation.

Chapter 5

Multiple Choice Questions:

1. C. Faculty salary scales
2. C. To ensure the program remains relevant and responsive to community health needs
3. B. NCLEX-RN pass rates
4. A. To identify gaps and ensure alignment with accreditation requirements
5. B. Learning Management Systems (LMS) and Student Information Systems (SIS)

True/False Questions:

1. True
2. False (Accreditation standards do require evidence of student support services)
3. True
4. False (Faculty must engage in ongoing professional development to maintain their expertise)
5. True

Short Answer Questions:

1. Curriculum design is critical because it must balance theoretical knowledge, clinical practice, and emerging trends, ensuring it meets national benchmarks like the AACN Essentials. An effective curriculum is essential for producing competent nurses and meeting accreditation standards related to content, delivery, and clinical preparation.
2. LMS and SIS help collect and analyze student performance data, track retention rates, and provide evidence for accreditation reviews. They streamline data reporting, making it easier to demonstrate compliance with accreditation standards related to student outcomes, program quality, and continuous improvement.
3. Challenges include outdated policies, lack of faculty involvement in policy revisions, and insufficient resources to implement changes. These can be overcome through a comprehensive policy audit, active collaboration among faculty and administrators, and clear communication regarding aligning policies with accreditation standards.
4. A clear and mission-driven statement aligns the program's goals with broader healthcare needs, ensuring that educational outcomes are focused on producing competent, culturally responsive nurses. It provides direction for curriculum development, faculty recruitment, and the establishment of student success metrics.

5. A program might use retention data to identify at-risk students early and offer tutoring, counseling, or mentorship. By proactively addressing the needs of at-risk students, programs can improve retention rates, as demonstrated in some programs where targeted interventions led to up to a 30% improvement in retention.

Discussion Questions:

1. Faculty qualifications are central to delivering quality nursing education. Accrediting bodies require nursing faculty to have advanced degrees and demonstrate ongoing professional development. Continuous faculty development ensures instructors remain up-to-date on clinical practices, evidence-based research, and new teaching methodologies, which ultimately enhances student learning and helps meet accreditation standards.
2. Programs can use data from student outcomes, faculty evaluations, and stakeholder feedback to identify areas for improvement. By regularly reviewing their curriculum, teaching methods, and student support services, programs can make data-driven adjustments to maintain accreditation compliance and enhance educational quality.
3. Aligning policies with accreditation standards ensures that the program is organized, well-resourced, and structured to meet educational and regulatory expectations. This alignment supports student success, enhances faculty development, and ensures that the program adheres to necessary quality benchmarks, all contributing to overall program effectiveness.
4. Student support services, such as academic advising, counseling, and clinical placement assistance, are vital in helping students succeed. Accreditation standards require programs to show how these services contribute to student outcomes. Effective student support can improve retention, graduation, and employment rates, which are key indicators of program success.
5. Programs in rural or underserved areas can build partnerships with local clinics and healthcare organizations to expand clinical placement opportunities. They could offer scholarships or mentorship programs to attract students from the community and improve access to nursing education. Tailoring programs to meet the specific healthcare needs of these communities would not only help meet accreditation standards and prepare graduates to address critical health disparities.

Chapter 6

1. **Answer:** Interpreting accreditation feedback is essential because it helps the program understand its strengths and areas needing improvement. It provides a clear roadmap for maintaining or achieving accreditation status. Programs should approach the feedback with a solution-oriented mindset, ensuring that all team members—faculty, administrators, and stakeholders—review the feedback thoroughly. They should prioritize feedback that addresses critical areas of non-compliance or significant improvement potential and develop action plans to address these issues.
2. **Answer:** Common recommendations include strengthening faculty development programs, improving clinical placements, enhancing student support services, and refining program outcomes assessments. These recommendations are vital because they highlight areas that directly affect student success, program quality, and the program's ability to meet accreditation standards. Addressing these areas can improve student retention, graduation rates, NCLEX pass rates, and overall program effectiveness.
3. **Answer:** The steps involved in developing an action plan include:

1. **Identifying deficiencies:** Review accreditation feedback and identify the specific areas that need improvement.
2. **Setting priorities:** Determine which issues are most critical and address them first.
3. **Assigning responsibilities:** Allocate tasks to staff members and faculty responsible for implementing changes.
4. **Developing timelines:** Set realistic deadlines for implementing changes and achieving goals.
5. **Evaluating progress:** Continuously monitor the effectiveness of implemented changes and make adjustments as needed. The critical elements include clear goals, timelines, responsible individuals, and measurable outcomes.

4. **Answer:** Nursing program administrators can communicate accreditation-related changes through regular meetings, emails, newsletters, and departmental briefings. Providing clear, written documentation outlining the changes and their implications is essential. Additionally, holding workshops or training sessions for faculty and staff can ensure that all parties understand how to implement the changes. For students, informational sessions or updated program handbooks can clarify the changes affecting their education.

5. **Answer:** Documenting improvements is essential for demonstrating that the program has addressed deficiencies and made progress toward meeting accreditation standards. The documentation should include evidence of the changes made (e.g., updated curricula, revised policies), data showing improvements (e.g., increased graduation rates or NCLEX pass rates), and feedback from stakeholders (e.g., faculty and student surveys). This documentation helps the accrediting agency assess the program's commitment to continuous improvement.

6. **Answer:** Strategies include establishing a culture of ongoing self-assessment, regularly collecting and analyzing data, and involving all stakeholders in decision-making. Programs should set up systems for continuous feedback (from students, faculty, and employers) and implement regular reviews of curricula, faculty development, and student outcomes. These strategies ensure that the program stays aligned with current healthcare needs, remains adaptable to changes, and continues to meet or exceed accreditation standards, contributing to long-term success.

7. **Answer:** Steps include:
   1. **Identifying key performance indicators (KPIs):** These could include student outcomes, faculty qualifications, clinical placements, and program evaluations.
   2. **Developing data collection systems:** Use tools like learning management systems (LMS) or student information systems (SIS) to gather relevant data.
   3. **Analyzing the data:** Look for trends like retention rates, student performance, and faculty development needs.
   4. **Making informed decisions:** Use the analysis to identify areas for improvement and allocate resources effectively. This data helps identify strengths, weaknesses, and trends, which can be used to guide improvements and meet accreditation standards.

8. **Answer:** Engaging faculty and staff can be done by forming committees to address specific feedback areas, holding regular meetings to review progress, and providing professional development opportunities aligned with accreditation standards. Best practices include recognizing and rewarding faculty contributions to the accreditation

process, fostering an environment of open communication, and ensuring faculty have a voice in decision-making processes related to program changes.

9. **Answer:** Prioritizing feedback ensures that the most critical areas impacting student success, program integrity, and compliance are addressed first. A program should evaluate deficiencies based on their severity and impact on accreditation standards. For example, issues related to faculty qualifications or clinical placement opportunities might have immediate consequences for accreditation. At the same time, less urgent matters, such as improving student satisfaction, could be addressed later.

2. **Answer:** Continuous self-reflection and assessment help the program stay proactive rather than reactive to accreditation feedback. By regularly evaluating program effectiveness, faculty performance, and student outcomes, the program can identify areas needing attention before they become problems. Practices to foster a culture of self-improvement include regularly scheduled program evaluations, feedback loops from stakeholders, and the integration of continuous quality improvement processes into the program's daily operations.

Chapter 7

Multiple Choice Questions

1. **B**. Complete re-evaluation of program faculty
2. **B**. Identify areas for program improvement
3. **B**. Every 3-5 years
4. **B**. Submission of periodic reports that show ongoing compliance
5. **B**. Enhances alignment with healthcare industry needs

True/False Questions

6. **True**
7. **False**
8. **False**
9. **False**
10. **True**

Short Answer Questions

11. The primary role of periodic reports in maintaining accreditation is to demonstrate that the nursing program continues to meet accreditation standards and showing evidence of improvements and compliance with previously identified recommendations.
12. The internal review process contributes to continuous quality improvement by regularly evaluating program outcomes, assessing gaps or areas of non-compliance, and implementing strategies for enhancement based on data-driven insights and stakeholder input.
13. It is important to involve key stakeholders because their perspectives ensure that the program is responsive to the needs of students, faculty, and the community. Their involvement also helps align program goals with industry demands, improving the overall quality and relevance of the education offered.
14. Common challenges include faculty turnover, maintaining an up-to-date curriculum, and resource constraints. These can be addressed by ensuring ongoing professional

development, regularly reviewing and updating curriculum based on industry trends, and seeking external funding or partnerships to support program resources.

15. Keeping up with changing accreditation standards ensures that nursing programs remain relevant, meet evolving healthcare needs, and maintain high education standards. This ongoing alignment allows the program to improve and serve students and the healthcare community better.

Essay Questions

16. A successful internal review process involves several key components: data collection, including student outcomes, NCLEX pass rates, and faculty feedback; stakeholder feedback, including input from students, faculty, and clinical partners; and faculty involvement in implementing improvements. Regular reviews help identify trends and challenges, allowing the program to address issues and ensure compliance with accreditation standards proactively.

17. To prepare for reaccreditation, nursing programs should start by reviewing feedback from previous accreditation cycles and conducting a self-study to identify areas for improvement. The program should collect and analyze relevant data, engage stakeholders for input, and address any recommendations or deficiencies. Building a clear action plan and ensuring that all faculty and staff are aligned with the program's goals will help demonstrate continuous improvement and commitment to high standards.

18. Nursing programs can maintain continuous quality improvement by regularly assessing program outcomes, collecting and analyzing student performance data, and adjusting curriculum and faculty development as needed. Technology can play a role in tracking and reporting outcomes efficiently while engaging stakeholders to ensure that improvements reflect the needs of both students and the healthcare community. Continuous professional development for faculty and a culture of ongoing evaluation is key to ensuring the program's success between accreditation cycles.

Chapter 8

1. **Common barriers** include financial constraints, staffing shortages, and resource limitations, which may hinder the ability of nursing programs to meet accreditation standards.

2. **To respond to non-compliance**, programs must first identify the areas of deficiency, develop a corrective action plan, implement changes, and provide evidence of improvements. Communication with accrediting bodies is essential to demonstrate progress and a commitment to compliance.

3. **Faculty turnover** is significant because it disrupts program stability and can affect program delivery. Strategies to minimize its impact include providing professional development opportunities, fostering faculty engagement, and ensuring that new faculty are properly onboarded.

4. **Leadership changes** can create instability and confusion during the accreditation process. To manage these transitions, programs should ensure continuity of leadership, delegate responsibilities, and communicate effectively with all stakeholders. Documenting progress and maintaining clear records is also crucial.

5. **External challenges** include changes in regulations, healthcare trends, and technological advancements. Nursing programs must remain flexible and adaptable, updating curricula and policies in response to these external shifts to ensure compliance with accreditation standards.

6. **Building resilience and adaptability** involves fostering a culture of continuous improvement, regularly reviewing program performance, engaging stakeholders in feedback loops, and staying current with industry trends. This allows programs to address challenges proactively.

7. **Leadership's role** in continuous improvement includes promoting a quality culture, ensuring regular evaluations, setting measurable goals, and prioritizing data-driven decisions. Engaging faculty and staff in the improvement process helps maintain a focus on long-term program success.

8. A **corrective action plan** outlines specific steps to address non-compliance, including identifying the issue, implementing changes, and setting timelines for improvement. Regular monitoring and documenting progress are key components of the plan.

9. **Stakeholder engagement** is crucial for maintaining accreditation because it ensures alignment between the program and its internal and external constituents. Programs should involve faculty, staff, students, administrators, and clinical partners in ongoing self-assessment and decision-making processes.

10. **Navigating changes in healthcare trends and regulations** requires a proactive approach. Nursing programs must continually review and revise their curricula, faculty development, and clinical placements to ensure alignment with the latest industry standards and regulatory requirements.

Chapter 9

11. Accreditation ensures that nursing programs meet established educational standards, guaranteeing quality and competency. It is important because it verifies that a program offers a curriculum that prepares students for professional practice, ensuring they meet the qualifications required for licensure.

12. Graduating from an accredited program increases a nurse's employability, as employers often require applicants to have graduated from an accredited institution. Accreditation is also necessary for students to qualify for federal financial aid and licensing exams, influencing their career prospects.

13. Accreditation ensures that nursing programs meet the standards required by state licensing boards. Graduates from accredited programs can sit for licensure exams (e.g., NCLEX-RN), which are essential for becoming a registered nurse. Without accreditation, graduates may not be able to pursue licensure.

14. Accreditation provides external validation that nursing programs adhere to rigorous educational standards. This assures the public, including potential students and employers, that the program produces competent, qualified nurses who can effectively provide high-quality care and contribute to healthcare settings.

15. Nursing programs can partner with hospitals, clinics, and healthcare systems to create clinical training opportunities that align with current healthcare practices. These collaborations help students gain hands-on experience, improve patient care, and ensure that students are well-prepared to meet industry demands while meeting accreditation standards.

16. Future trends may include a greater emphasis on interprofessional education, integrating technology such as telemedicine, and adapting curricula to address evolving healthcare needs (e.g., geriatrics and mental health). These trends will ensure that nursing education stays relevant and that nurses are prepared for new challenges in healthcare.

17. Accreditation standards influence nursing curricula by ensuring they are comprehensive, up-to-date, and aligned with healthcare needs. Programs must continually evaluate and adjust their curriculum to meet accreditation requirements, leading to high-quality education that prepares students to excel in nursing.

18. Accredited programs help create a highly qualified nursing workforce directly linked to improved patient outcomes. Studies have shown that nurses in accredited programs are better equipped with the skills to provide high-quality, evidence-based care, ultimately improving patient safety and satisfaction.

19. If a nursing program loses its accreditation, it can no longer offer graduates the opportunity to sit for licensure exams, and students may not be eligible for federal financial aid. This can lead to a loss of reputation, a decrease in enrollment, and financial instability for the program.

20. Program evaluation is essential for assessing whether nursing programs meet accreditation standards and whether they are continuously improving. Through regular evaluations, programs can identify areas for improvement, implement necessary changes, and ensure compliance with accreditation requirements, which is essential for ongoing success.

References By Chapter

Chapter 1

Accreditation Commission for Education in Nursing (ACEN). (2020). *ACEN Annual Report.* Retrieved from www.acenursing.org

American Association of Colleges of Nursing (AACN). (2021). *The Impact of Accreditation on Nursing Education.* Retrieved from www.aacnnursing.org

National Council of State Boards of Nursing (NCBSN). (2020). *National Licensing Examination Pass Rates by Program Type.* Retrieved from www.ncsbn.org

National League for Nursing (NLN). (2021). *Hiring Preferences and Accreditation: Employers' Perspective.* Retrieved from www.nln.org

U.S. Bureau of Labor Statistics (BLS). (2021). *Registered Nurses: Employment Projections.* Retrieved from www.bls.gov

Chapter 2

Accreditation Commission for Education in Nursing (2023). *Standards and Criteria for Accreditation.*

Commission on Collegiate Nursing Education (2022). *Accreditation Handbook.*

National League for Nursing (2021). *Survey of Accreditation Trends.*

Quality and Safety Education for Nurses (2022). *Competencies for Nursing Education.*

U.S. Department of Education (2023). *Recognized Accrediting Bodies and Standards.*

American Journal of Nursing (2021). "Achieving Excellence in Nursing Accreditation."

Miller, M., & Jafar, H. (2019). *Quality Assurance and Accreditation in Nursing Education: A Global Perspective.* Journal of Clinical Nursing, 28(11-12), 2171-2179. https://doi.org/10.1111/jocn.14801

American Nurses Association (ANA). (2020). *The Value of Accreditation in Nursing Education.* Retrieved from https://www.nursingworld.org

Schmidt, N. A., & Brown, J. M. (2021). *Evidence-Based Practice for Nurses: Appraisal and Application of Research.* Elsevier Health Sciences.

Stokowski, L. A. (2018). *Preparing for Accreditation: Key Steps and Lessons Learned from Schools of Nursing.* Journal of Nursing Education, 57(5), 261-267. https://doi.org/10.3928/01484834-20180420-01

National Council of State Boards of Nursing (NCSBN). (2021). *The NCLEX-RN Examination: A Guide to the Licensing Process for Nurses.* Retrieved from https://www.ncsbn.org

Council for Higher Education Accreditation (CHEA). (2020). *The Role of Accreditation in Higher Education.*

Retrieved from https://www.chea.org

U.S. Department of Education. (2022). *Accreditation in the United States.* Retrieved from https://www.ed.gov/accreditation

National League for Nursing (NLN). (2021). *Accreditation and the Role of the NLN Commission for Nursing Education Accreditation.* Retrieved from https://www.nln.org

Commission on Collegiate Nursing Education (CCNE). (2021). *Standards for Accreditation of Baccalaureate and Graduate Nursing Programs.* Washington, DC: American Association of Colleges of Nursing.

American Association of Colleges of Nursing (AACN). (2020). *Accreditation: The Pathway to Program Excellence.* Retrieved from https://www.aacnnursing.org

Chapter 3

Accreditation Commission for Education in Nursing (ACEN). (2021). *Standards and criteria for accreditation of nursing programs.* Retrieved from https://www.acenursing.org

American Association of Colleges of Nursing (AACN). (2020). *The Essentials: Core Competencies for Professional Nursing Education.* Retrieved from https://www.aacnnursing.org

National League for Nursing (NLN). (2019). *Accreditation Manual for Nursing Education Programs.* National League for Nursing.

Barker, K., & Hutton, C. (Eds.) (2017). *Accreditation for Allied Health Programs: A Guide for Educators and Administrators.* Springer Publishing.

Campbell, S. L., & McLean, M. R. (2019). *Curriculum development and accreditation in nursing education.* Journal of Nursing Education, 58(4), 209-214. https://doi.org/10.3928/01484834-20190321-03

Jeffries, P. R. (2016). *Simulation in Nursing Education: From Conceptualization to Evaluation.* Springer Publishing.

Luzinski, T. R., & Capelle, L. M. (2018). *Assessment and accreditation: The changing landscape of nursing education.* Journal of Nursing Education, 57(5), 276-282. https://doi.org/10.3928/01484834-20180423-02

Oermann, M. H., & Gaberson, K. B. (2018). *Evaluation and Testing in Nursing Education.* Springer Publishing.

Spector, N., & Kappel, M. (Eds.) (2019). *Nursing Education: A Conceptual Approach to Teaching and Learning.* Wiley-Blackwell.

U.S. Department of Education. (2020). *Accrediting Agencies: Information and Standards for Higher Education Institutions.* Retrieved from https://www.ed.gov/accreditation

Chapter 4

Accreditation Commission for Education in Nursing (ACEN). (2020). *Accreditation Manual.* Accreditation Commission for

Education in Nursing. Retrieved from www.acenursing.org

American Association of Colleges of Nursing (AACN). (2021). *Essentials of Baccalaureate Education for Professional Nursing Practice.* American Association of Colleges of Nursing. Retrieved from www.aacnnursing.org

Hutchinson, M., & Jackson, D. (2017). *The Role of Site Visits in Accreditation: Best Practices and Recommendations.* Journal of Nursing Education, 56(6), 353-359. https://doi.org/10.3928/01484834-20170516-04

National League for Nursing (NLN). (2019). *Accreditation of Nursing Programs: Standards and Guidelines for Accreditation of Baccalaureate and Graduate Nursing Programs.* National League for Nursing. Retrieved from www.nln.org

American Nurses Association (ANA). (2015). *The Nursing Professional Development Specialist's Guide to Accreditation: Achieving Compliance and Sustaining Excellence.* American Nurses Association.

Kusumoto, T., & Yamamoto, K. (2021). *Preparing for Site Visits in Nursing Education Accreditation.* Journal of Clinical Nursing Education, 10(3), 45-56. https://doi.org/10.1007/jcne.2021.03

Council for Higher Education Accreditation (CHEA). (2020). *Understanding the Accreditation Process: A Guide for Faculty, Staff, and Administrators.* Council for Higher

Education Accreditation. Retrieved from www.chea.org

White, L., & McClain, J. (2018). *Accreditation and Site Visits: Navigating the Challenges in Nursing Programs.* Nurse Educator, 43(1), 31-36. https://doi.org/10.1097/NNE.0000000000000437

Carnegie Foundation for the Advancement of Teaching. (2020). *Assessment and Accreditation: Key Insights from Higher Education Experts.* Carnegie Foundation for the Advancement of Teaching. Retrieved from www.carnegiefoundation.org

Barger, S., & Decker, J. (2021). *Preparing for Accreditation Site Visits in Health Care Education Programs.* Journal of Allied Health, 50(2), 79-85. https://doi.org/10.1016/j.jah.2021.01.002

Association of Colleges of Nursing Education (ACNE). (2022). *Guidelines for Effective Site Visits: What Accreditation Teams Look for.* Association of Colleges of Nursing Education. Retrieved from www.acne.org

Chapter 5

Accreditation Commission for Education in Nursing (ACEN). (2022). *Standards and Criteria for Nursing Program Accreditation.* Retrieved from https://www.acenursing.org

American Association of Colleges of Nursing (AACN). (2021). *The Essentials: Core Competencies for Professional Nursing Education.*

Retrieved from https://www.aacnnursing.org

National League for Nursing (NLN). (2020). *NLN Accreditation Standards and Criteria.* Retrieved from https://www.nln.org

National Council of State Boards of Nursing (NCSBN). (2021). *NCLEX-RN Examination: Annual Report.* Retrieved from https://www.ncsbn.org

U.S. Department of Education (ED). (2020). *Accreditation in the United States: Requirements and Process.* Retrieved from https://www.ed.gov

National Center for Education Statistics (NCES). (2021). *Integrated Postsecondary Education Data System (IPEDS): Nursing Programs and Outcomes.* Retrieved from https://nces.ed.gov

Schmidt, N. A., & Brown, J. M. (2021). *Evidence-Based Practice for Nurses: Appraisal and Application of Research.* Jones & Bartlett Learning.

White, K. M., & Dudley-Brown, S. (2020). *Translation of Evidence into Nursing and Healthcare.* Springer Publishing Company.

Wolf, L., & Fagan, D. (2019). *An Overview of the Role of Accreditation in Nursing Education: Standards, Challenges, and Best Practices.* Journal of Nursing Education, 58(9), 504-511.

Jones, C. B., & Bell, M. M. (2020). *Nursing Program Evaluation: Tools and Techniques for Continuous Improvement.* Springer Publishing.

Buerhaus, P. I., Skinner, L. E., Auerbach, D. I., & Staiger, D. O. (2020). *The Impact of Nursing Education on the Nursing Workforce: Challenges and Opportunities.* Journal of Nursing Administration, 50(7-8), 391-399.

Chapter 6

Accreditation Commission for Education in Nursing (ACEN). (2017). *Accreditation Manual for Nursing Programs.* Retrieved from www.acenursing.org.

American Association of Colleges of Nursing (AACN). (2020). *The Essentials of Baccalaureate Education for Professional Nursing Practice.* Retrieved from www.aacnnursing.org.

National League for Nursing (NLN). (2018). *NLN Accreditation Standards for Nursing Education Programs.* Retrieved from www.nln.org.

National Council of State Boards of Nursing (NCSBN). (2021). *NCLEX-RN Examination Statistics.* Retrieved from www.ncsbn.org.

Commission on Collegiate Nursing Education (CCNE). (2020). *Standards for Accreditation of Baccalaureate and Graduate Nursing Programs.* Retrieved from www.aacnnursing.org/CCNE.

Watson, C. (2019). *Managing Accreditation: A Guide for Nursing Programs.* New York, NY: Springer Publishing Company.

Peden, M., & Bowers, J. (2018). *Addressing Deficiencies in Nursing Programs: The Role of Accreditation Feedback.* Journal of Nursing

Education and Practice, 8(4), 112-118.

Clark, R., & Jackson, S. (2020). *Sustaining Improvement in Nursing Programs: Best Practices for Continuous Quality Assurance.* Journal of Nursing Accreditation, 10(2), 79-86. https://doi.org/10.1080/0098138X.2020.1728902

Thompson, D. (2017). *Accreditation and Program Improvement in Nursing Education: Strategies for Responding to Feedback.* Nursing Education Perspectives, 38(3), 157-162. https://doi.org/10.1097/01.NEP.0000000000000205

Bender, M., & Williams, P. (2016). *Building a Culture of Continuous Improvement in Nursing Education Programs.* Journal of Nursing Administration, 46(7-8), 350-356. https://doi.org/10.1097/NNA.0000000000000390

Chapter 7

Accreditation Commission for Education in Nursing (ACEN). (2021). *ACEN Accreditation Standards and Criteria for Nursing Programs.* Retrieved from www.acenursing.org

American Association of Colleges of Nursing (AACN). (2020). *The Essentials of Baccalaureate Education for Professional Nursing Practice.* Washington, DC: AACN.

National League for Nursing (NLN). (2022). *Accreditation Manual for Nursing Education Programs.* Retrieved from www.nln.org

Council for Higher Education Accreditation (CHEA). (2021). *Accreditation and Quality Assurance in Higher Education.* Retrieved from www.chea.org

National Council of State Boards of Nursing (NCSBN). (2022). *Nursing Education Accreditation and Continuing Education Guide.* Retrieved from www.ncsbn.org

Harris, M., & Smith, J. (2019). *Effective Strategies for Maintaining Accreditation in Nursing Education.* Journal of Nursing Education, 58(3), 123-130. https://doi.org/10.3928/01484834-20190212-04

Sullivan, M. E. (2020). *Continuous Quality Improvement and Accreditation: A Nursing Perspective.* Nursing Education Perspectives, 41(1), 45-52. https://doi.org/10.1097/01.NEP.0000000000000567

Haddad, L., & Kelly, M. (2019). *The Role of Data in Sustaining Nursing Program Accreditation.* Journal of Nursing Administration, 49(7-8), 379-384. https://doi.org/10.1097/NNA.0000000000000792

American Association of Colleges of Nursing (AACN). (2018). *Strategies for Ensuring Success in Reaccreditation of Nursing Programs.* Journal of Nursing Education, 57(2), 63-69. https://doi.org/10.3928/01484834-20180124-02

Hughes, J., & Anderson, T. (2020). *Stakeholder Engagement in the Continuous Improvement of Nursing Education Programs.* International Journal of Nursing Education Scholarship, 17(1), 12-22.

https://doi.org/10.1515/ijnes-2020-0020

Chapter 8

American Association of Colleges of Nursing (AACN). (2020). *Nursing Faculty Shortage Fact Sheet.* Retrieved from www.aacnnursing.org.

National Council of State Boards of Nursing (NCSBN). (2021). *National Council Licensure Examination (NCLEX) for Registered Nurses Pass Rates.* Retrieved from www.ncsbn.org.

National Nursing Workforce Survey. (2021). *Trends in the U.S. Nursing Workforce: Insights into Retention and Mobility.*

U.S. Bureau of Labor Statistics (BLS). (2021). *Registered Nurses: Occupational Outlook Handbook.* Retrieved from www.bls.gov.

National Center for Healthcare Workforce Analysis. (2021). *Addressing Workforce Shortages and Resource Gaps in Healthcare Education and Training.* U.S. Department of Health and Human Services.

Journal of Nursing Education. (2020). *Barriers to Accreditation Compliance in Nursing Programs: Insights from Recent Case Studies.* Retrieved from www.journalofnursingeducation.com.

Council for Higher Education Accreditation (CHEA). (2020). *Strategies for Overcoming Common Accreditation Barriers.* Retrieved from www.chea.org.

Accreditation Commission for Education in Nursing (ACEN). (2019). *Guidelines for Addressing Accreditation Deficiencies in Nursing Programs.* Retrieved from www.acenursing.org.

Healthcare Workforce Report. (2021). *Improving the Accreditation Process for Nursing Programs: Trends and Recommendations.*

Chapter 9

American Association of Colleges of Nursing (AACN). (2020). *Impact of Accreditation on Nursing Education and Practice.* Retrieved from www.aacnnursing.org.

National Council of State Boards of Nursing (NCSBN). (2021). *The Role of Accreditation in Ensuring NCLEX-RN Success Rates.* Retrieved from www.ncsbn.org.

National League for Nursing (NLN). (2020). *Accreditation and the Advancement of Nursing Education: A Comprehensive Overview.* Retrieved from www.nln.org.

Journal of Nursing Education. (2021). *How Accreditation Influences Employment Opportunities and Career Advancement for Nursing Graduates.* Retrieved from www.journalofnursingeducation.com.

U.S. Department of Health and Human Services (HHS). (2021). *Accreditation's Impact on Workforce Development and Public Health Initiatives.* Retrieved from www.hhs.gov.

National Center for Healthcare Workforce Analysis. (2021). *The Future of Nursing: Advancing Education* *and Healthcare through Accreditation.* Retrieved from www.hrsa.gov.

Healthcare Education Association (HEA). (2020). *Improving Healthcare Outcomes through Nursing Program Accreditation.* Retrieved from www.healthcareeducationassociation.org.

Council for Higher Education Accreditation (CHEA). (2020). *Accreditation and Its Role in Promoting Public Confidence in Nursing Programs.* Retrieved from www.chea.org.

World Health Organization (WHO). (2021). *Global Health Workforce: The Role of Nursing and Accreditation in Advancing Education.* Retrieved from www.who.int.

American Nurses Association (ANA). (2020). *How Accreditation Enhances Public Trust in Nursing Programs and Healthcare Education.* Retrieved from www.nursingworld.org.

Chapter 10

Accreditation Commission for Education in Nursing (ACEN). (n.d.). *Accreditation Standards and Criteria.* Retrieved from https://www.acenursing.org/

Society for Simulation in Healthcare (SSH). (n.d.). *Accreditation Standards for Simulation Programs.* Retrieved from https://www.ssih.org/

National Board of Certification and Recertification for Nurse Anesthetists (NBCRNA). (2023). *Certification Process and Requirements for*

Nurse Anesthetists. Retrieved from https://www.nbcrna.com/

Council on Accreditation of Nurse Anesthesia Educational Programs (COA). (2020). *Accreditation Standards for Nurse Anesthesia Programs.* Retrieved from https://www.coa.us.com/

National League for Nursing (NLN). (2021). *Accreditation of Nursing Programs.* Retrieved from https://www.nln.org/

American Association of Colleges of Nursing (AACN). (2021). *The Essentials: Core Competencies for Professional Nursing Education.* Retrieved from https://www.aacnnursing.org/

American Association of Nurse Anesthetists (AANA). (2022). *Nurse Anesthesia Programs and Accreditation Standards.* Retrieved from https://www.aana.com/

Baker, S., & Stanley, M. (2019). *Simulation in Nursing Education: From Theory to Practice.* New York, NY: Springer Publishing.

Clark, D. (2018). *The Role of Simulation in Enhancing Nursing Education: A Review of Accreditation Standards. Journal of Nursing Education,* 57(9), 514-520. https://doi.org/10.3928/01484834-20180822-03

Sullivan, S. R., & Vick, D. J. (2020). *Implementing Simulation in Nurse Anesthesia Programs: Challenges and Best Practices. Nurse Educator,* 45(2), 89-94. https://doi.org/10.1097/NNE.0000000000000800

Tanner, C. A. (2019). *Simulation in Nursing Education: A Comprehensive Review. Nursing Education Perspectives,* 40(5), 267-273. https://doi.org/10.1097/01.NEP.0 00000000000559

Institute of Medicine (IOM). (2011). *The Future of Nursing: Leading Change, Advancing Health.* Washington, D.C.: National Academy Press. Retrieved from https://www.ncbi.nlm.nih.gov/boo ks/NBK20988/

National Council of State Boards of Nursing (NCSBN). (2021). *The Impact of Simulation in Nursing Education and the NCLEX-RN Exam.* Retrieved from https://www.ncsbn.org/

International Nursing Association for Clinical Simulation and Learning (INACSL). (2021). *Standards of Best Practice: Simulation. Clinical Simulation in Nursing,* 53, 20-24. https://doi.org/10.1016/j.ecns.202 1.04.004

Yoder, L. H. (2018). *The Influence of Accreditation on Nursing Education and Practice. Nursing Outlook,* 66(4), 347-353. https://doi.org/10.1016/j.outlook.2 018.03.003

NCLEX Statistics and Reports. Retrieved from https://www.ncsbn.org

National Center for Education Statistics (NCES). (2022). *Integrated Postsecondary Education Data System (IPEDS).* Retrieved from https://nces.ed.gov/ipeds/

Accreditation Commission for Education in Nursing (ACEN). (2022). *Accreditation Standards and Criteria.* Retrieved from https://www.acenursing.org

Journal of Nursing Education. Various articles on program evaluation, faculty development, and retention strategies. Retrieved from https://www.healio.com/nursing/j ournals/jne

National League for Nursing (NLN). (2021). *Transforming Nursing Education: Leading the Call to Reform.* Retrieved from https://www.nln.org

Thomas, K., & Quinlan, C. (2020). *Quality Assurance in Nursing Education.* Nursing Outlook, 68(4), 342–348.

U.S. Department of Education. (2022). *Guidelines for Accrediting Agencies and Postsecondary Institutions.* Retrieved from https://www.ed.gov/accreditation

Berkow, S., Virkstis, K., Stewart, J., & Conway, L. (2022). *Assessing Student Outcomes in Nursing Education.* Nurse Educator Today, 102, 50-55.

Appendix A

American Association of Colleges of Nursing (AACN). (2021). *The Essentials: Core Competencies for Professional Nursing Education.* Retrieved from https://www.aacnnursing.org

National Council of State Boards of Nursing (NCSBN). (2023).

Appendix B

American Association of Colleges of Nursing (AACN). (2021).

Guidelines for Governance in Nursing Education.

Accreditation Commission for Education in Nursing (ACEN). (2022). *Accreditation Standards and Criteria.*

National League for Nursing (NLN). (2020). *Best Practices in Shared Governance.*

Appendix C

American Association of Colleges of Nursing (AACN). (2021). *Guidelines for Governance in Nursing Education.*

Accreditation Commission for Education in Nursing (ACEN). (2022). *Accreditation Standards and Criteria.*

National League for Nursing (NLN). (2020). *Best Practices in Shared Governance.*

Appendix D

Accreditation Commission for Education in Nursing (ACEN). (2022). *Standards and Criteria for Curriculum Assessment.*

American Association of Colleges of Nursing (AACN). (2021). *The Essentials of Baccalaureate Education for Professional Nursing Practice.*

National League for Nursing (NLN). (2020). *Curriculum Innovation in Nursing Education.*

Smith, J. & Jones, R. (2019). *Best Practices in Curriculum Design for Nursing Programs. Journal of Nursing Education,* 58(4), 245-252.

Appendix E

Accreditation Commission for Education in Nursing (ACEN). (2022). *Standards for Nursing Education Facilities.*

American Association of Colleges of Nursing (AACN). (2021). *Facility Guidelines for Nursing Programs.*

National League for Nursing (NLN). (2020). *Optimizing Nursing Education Spaces.*

Brown, T., & Carter, L. (2021). *Advancing Nursing Education Through Technology and Facility Design. Journal of Nursing Education,* 60(3), 145-150.

Appendix F

Accreditation Commission for Education in Nursing (ACEN). (2022). *Standards and Criteria for Nursing Program Staffing.*

American Association of Colleges of Nursing (AACN). (2021). *Guidelines for Faculty Workload and Qualifications.*

Smith, A., & Johnson, P. (2021). *Effective Staffing Models in Nursing Education. Journal of Nursing Education,* 60(4), 210-215.

National League for Nursing (NLN). (2020). *Ensuring Adequate Staffing in Nursing Programs.*

List of Figures

Upcoming from this author

Simulation Operation in Healthcare Education: A primer into the role of Operations in Medical and Nursing Training

Mastering Healthcare Management and Operations: Insights, case studies, and practical strategies

Strategic Healthcare Simulation: Operations, Planning, and Alignment with Accreditation Standards.

Incorporating the ADDIE Instructional Design Model in Healthcare Simulation Curriculum

Exercise and Evaluation: Combining Healthcare Simulation and the Hospital Incident Command System (HICS)

Available Now!

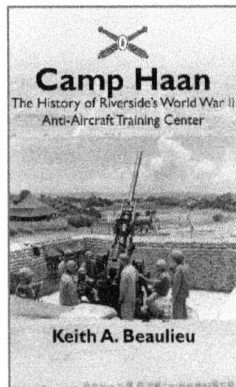

Camp Haan
The History of Riverside's World War II
Anti-Aircraft Training Center

Keith A. Beaulieu

amazon

BARNES&NOBLE
BOOKSELLERS

IngramSpark

www.ingramcontent.com/pod-product-compliance
Lightning Source LLC
Chambersburg PA
CBHW081155020426

42333CB00020B/2511